HEARING IMPAIRMENTS IN YOUNG CHILDREN

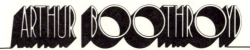

ARTHUR BOOTHROYD

The Clarke School for the Deaf

HEARING IMPAIRMENTS IN YOUNG CHILDREN

Prentice-Hall, Inc., Englewood Cliffs, N.J. 07632

Library of Congress Cataloging in Publication Data

BOOTHROYD, ARTHUR.
    Hearing impairments in young children.

    (Remediation of communication disorders)
    Bibliography: p.
    Includes index.
    1. Hearing disorders in children. 2. Children,
Deaf—Rehabilitation. I. Title. II. Series.
[DNLM: 1. Hearing disorders—In infancy and child-
hood. 2. Hearing disorders—Therapy. WV 271 B725h]
RF291.5.C45B66   618.92'09789   618.92'29789   81-5915
ISBN 0-13-3847012   AACR2

© 1982 by Prentice-Hall, Inc., Englewood Cliffs, N.J. 07632

TO JOHN, ANDREW, AND PETER

618.9209789
B725h

Printed in the United States of America

10 9 8 7 6 5 4 3 2 1

Editorial/production supervision by Virginia Cavanagh Neri
Interior design by Maureen Olsen
Cover design by Maureen Olsen
Manufacturing buyer: Edmund W. Leone
Photographs and artwork by Arthur Boothroyd

Prentice-Hall International, Inc., *London*
Prentice-Hall of Australia Pty. Limited, *Sydney*
Prentice-Hall of Canada, Ltd., *Toronto*
Prentice-Hall of India Private Limited, *New Delhi*
Prentice-Hall of Japan, Inc., *Tokyo*
Prentice-Hall of Southeast Asia Pte. Ltd., *Singapore*
Whitehall Books Limited, *Wellington, New Zealand*

210876

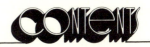

CONTENTS

Statement of the problem 1

Normal hearing 12

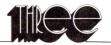

Child development and normal hearing 24

Impaired hearing 41

Development of the hearing impaired child 57

Goals and components of management 72

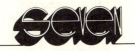

Audiological management 78

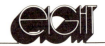

Auditory management 96

Cognitive and linguistic management 115

Speech management 145

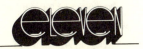

Parental management 171

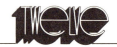

Social and emotional management 180

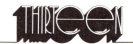

Special cases 186

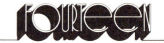

Delivery 200

Appendix 213

References 226

Index 231

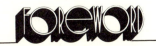

With the information explosion of recent years there has been a proliferation of knowledge in the areas of scientific and social inquiry. The speciality of communicative disorders has been no exception. While two decades ago a single textbook or "handbook" might have sufficed to provide the aspiring or practicing clinician with enlightenment on an array of communication handicaps, this is no longer possible—hence the decision to prepare a series of single-author texts.

As the title implies, the emphasis of this series, *Remediation of Communication Disorders,* is on therapy and treatment. The authors of each book were asked to provide information relative to anatomical and physiological aspects of each disorder, as well as pathology, etiology, and diagnosis to the extent that an understanding of these factors bears on management procedures. In such relatively short books this was quite a challenge: to offer guidance without writing a "cookbook"; to be selective without being parochial; to offer theory without losing sight of practice. To this challenge the series' authors have risen magnificently.

For all the reasons that an author is chosen to write a book in a speciality area like the management of young hearing-impaired children, Arthur Boothroyd is uniquely qualified. It was as a parent of a hearing-impaired child that he was introduced to this field, and in this role he first worked with Sir Alexander and Lady Ethel Ewing at the University of Manchester. His degree in physics provides a knowledge of the acoustical aspects of audiology, his four years of experience as a classroom teacher of children with normal hearing allows for the special insights accorded to few audiologists, and his more than twenty years of experience as a clinical audiologist have provided him with background in all aspects of the management of hearing-impaired children. Dr. Boothroyd's ability to take information from a variety of fields and to synthesize it in logical and meaningful ways is enhanced by his outstanding research, his background as a musician (he is an accomplished pianist), and his interest in the psychological, esthetic, and communicative aspects of audition. As director of the parent-infant and preschool programs at the Clarke School for the Deaf, Dr. Boothroyd's reputation is far reaching. The global approach taken in this book will surely make it a classic.

FREDERICK N. MARTIN
Series Editor

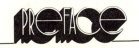

The topic of this book is *early intervention*—doing things that otherwise would not be done in order to change the course of development of young children. Development is influenced by many factors. These include innate capacities, inner drives, maturation, external pressures, parental input, parental responses, and so on. The intact child in a healthy family environment progresses smoothly and in synchrony with him or herself and with the surroundings. Needs, skills, and abilities develop in step with one another, thus providing mutual reinforcement. Parent and child meet each other's evolving needs and again provide mutual reinforcement. All aspects of development favor the emergence of a competent, independent adult.

When the child's sense of hearing is absent or defective, development follows a different course. Needs, skills, and abilities emerge at different rates; parent and child fail to meet each other's evolving needs; and mutual reinforcement is often replaced by mutual interference. Without intervention, the end result is a dependent adult lacking in emotional, social, communicative and intellectual competence. In a responsible, caring society, such an outcome is intolerable. Experience has shown that it is also unnecessary. By timely, appropriate intervention we can redirect the course of development and realize the human potential of the hearing-impaired child.

It is, of course, much easier to advocate early intervention than to implement it successfully. This kind of work requires professionals whose attributes include knowledge from several disciplines, the ability to synthesize this knowledge and apply it to real-life situations, the sensitivity and flexibility to adapt to the differing needs of individuals, the ability to establish rapport with children and with parents in crisis, and the emotional integrity needed to foster independence in others. It could justifiably be argued that any teacher or therapist needs these qualities, but young hearing-impaired children and their families are particularly dependent on professional help and therefore particularly vulnerable to professional shortcomings. Unfortunately, the training of early intervention specialists has not kept pace with demand, and management responsibility must often be assigned to persons with inadequate theoretical backgrounds and little or no supervised experience.

It is to the practitioner that this book is primarily addressed. My goal has been to provide a comprehensive view of the problem and to show how the multiple needs of hearing-impaired children and their families can be met within the constraints of practical intervention programs. This approach

should also be of value to students of communication disorders and education of the deaf, teacher educators, allied professionals, and parents.

The skills of early intervention cannot be acquired simply by reading
books. A book can offer new information and new perspectives, but the
assimilation of this input and its incorporation into professional development must be orchestrated from within. It must also be supported by practical experience — preferably under the supervision of a master teacher.
Keeping these limitations in mind I have tried to steer a middle road between "cookbook" and "treatise," and to offer a conceptual framework
supported by practical guidelines. In the process I have drawn from the
work of many people whose names will be found in the lists of reading
suggestions at the ends of the chapters.

One cannot write for long on the subject of childhood hearing impairment without confronting the issue of language modality. This issue has
polarized educators of the deaf for many years and will doubtless continue
to do so. At one extreme are those who see mastery of spoken language as
the only key to successful intervention and pursue this goal with single
minded determination. At the other are those who respond to the child's
emerging needs by providing a more accessible language system in which
speech is supplemented by manual signs. In fact, neither approach offers a
simple solution and there is no method of intervention that can be applied
to all children with uniform effectiveness. Implicit in this text is an approach
that considers all of the variables and needs impinging on a particular case
and develops goals, priorities, and procedures accordingly.

○ ACKNOWLEDGMENTS

Numerous past and present colleagues have contributed directly or
indirectly to these pages. They include Sir Alexander and Lady Ethel Ewing,
Ian Taylor, Gordon Campbell, Angela Broomfield-Foulkes, Dale Wilson,
Nancy Poland, and Nancy Hoar. I am particularly grateful to my friend and
colleague, Janice Gatty, who not only taught me most of what I know about
child development but was always willing to listen to first drafts and to
provide encouragement. The bulk of the manuscript was typed by Sheila
Paget and the project seen through to completion by Joyce Tutun. George
Pratt and the Board of Trustees of the Clarke School for the Deaf provided
both moral and material support. My best teachers have always been the
children with whom I have worked, and the best of all has been my hearing-
impaired son, Peter. To all of these I offer my sincere thanks. In a very real
sense this book is theirs. (I wish it were so easy to relinquish responsibility
for the errors.)

Arthur Boothroyd

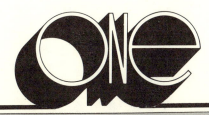

Statement of the problem

We live in a sea of air. Anything that moves must therefore disturb the air around it. Because air is an elastic medium, disturbances at one place are carried to other places in the form of waves—much as a pebble thrown into a pond causes ripples to spread over the surface. If these waves are capable of stimulating the sense of hearing, we call them *sound.* Sound travels very quickly (about 1,000 feet in a second) and therefore provides a timely source of information about movements occurring elsewhere. *Hearing* is what happens when we detect and interpret sounds. It permits us to perceive events at a distance.

At a primitive level of evolution, hearing is a simple survival mechanism. Animals use hearing to locate food and to avoid becoming someone else's food. At a more advanced level, hearing is used for communication. Animals generate sound patterns to produce specific behaviors in other animals. In man, this use of sound for communication has become very sophisticated. The sounds of speech serve as a medium for *language*—a system of symbols used for exchanging conceptually organized thoughts. Spoken language makes possible complex social interactions and, together with its written derivative, is one of the foundations of civilization.

Most children acquire spoken language skills during the first few years of life. They do so effortlessly and without formal instruction. All they require is the chance to interact regularly with people who already use spoken language. But some children have hearing impairments. That is to say, they have difficulty detecting sounds, interpreting sounds, or both. Such children are denied full access to the sound patterns of speech, both their own and other people's. The spontaneous acquisition of spoken language is therefore impeded or prevented. Unless this problem is resolved, the long term consequences are severe and wide ranging.

○ DEFINITION OF TERMS

Please note the generic use of the term *hearing impairment.* I am using this term to include all disorders of hearing, regardless of their nature, cause, or severity.

There are two major subgroups of hearing impairment—hearing loss and auditory processing disorder. A *hearing loss* is an impairment of sound detection. It can be measured in terms of the number of decibels by which the threshold of hearing is raised above normal. Descriptive labels are often attached, such as mild, moderate, severe, profound, and total. There is, however, a lack of agreement among professionals regarding the proper use of these qualifiers. The second type of hearing impairment—an *auditory processing disorder*—is an impairment of sound interpretation. Such disorders originate in the neural mechanism of hearing and may be caused by direct physical damage or by improper development. It is not uncommon for a given child to exhibit both a hearing loss *and* an auditory processing disorder.

Two other terms in popular use are *deaf* and *hard-of-hearing.* These terms have had an uncomfortable history since accepted definitions have repeatedly been made obsolete by increased knowledge and improved treatment. I suggest that they should be used to describe how an individual uses hearing (with amplification, if necessary), as follows:

Hard-of-hearing An adjective describing a person whose hearing, though impaired, is used as the primary modality for speech perception and acquisition.

Deaf An adjective describing a person whose hearing is not used as the primary modality for speech perception and acquisition, though it may be used as a supplement to vision or touch.

Totally deaf An adjective describing a subgroup of deaf persons who are without a sense of hearing or whose hearing is so rudimentary or so poorly developed as to be of no assistance in the perception and acquisition of speech. Another adjective for such persons is *nonauditory.*

For ease of reference, these definitions are summarized in Figure 1–1.

○ CONSEQUENCES OF HEARING IMPAIRMENT

Because of the complex nature of human development, a primary impairment of hearing will, if left untreated, cause several secondary impairments. To illustrate the process by which this occurs, consider those children with congenital hearing losses severe enough to prevent them from hearing speech, both their own and other people's. Assume further that the parents of these children are normally hearing and have not previously encountered hearing-impaired people. (And remember also that we are assuming no professional intervention.) What begins as a sensory problem becomes

1. *A perceptual problem* The children cannot identify objects and events by the sounds they make.

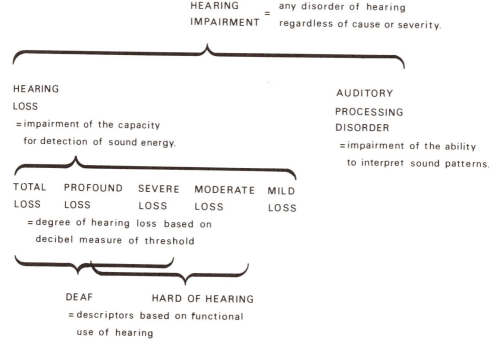

HEARING   = any disorder of hearing
IMPAIRMENT   regardless of cause or severity.

HEARING
LOSS
= impairment of the capacity
   for detection of sound energy.

AUDITORY
PROCESSING
DISORDER
= impairment of the ability
   to interpret sound patterns.

TOTAL   PROFOUND   SEVERE   MODERATE   MILD
LOSS   LOSS   LOSS   LOSS   LOSS
= degree of hearing loss based on
   decibel measure of threshold

DEAF   HARD OF HEARING
= descriptors based on functional
   use of hearing

FIGURE 1–1 Classification of hearing impairments and definitions of terms. Note that there has been little standardization of terminology related to hearing impairments and that usage in this text may be different from that in other texts. See Chapter Four for further information on degree of hearing loss.

2. *A speech problem* The children do not learn the connection between the movements of their speech mechanisms and the resulting sounds. Consequently, they do not acquire control of speech.

3. *A communication problem* The children do not learn their native language. They cannot, therefore, express thoughts to other people except by gesture or other concrete acts; they cannot understand what people say to them; and they cannot participate in conversational exchange.

4. *A cognitive problem* Children with language have access to their world through the minds of other people, through abstract ideas, and through information about distant times and distant places. Children without language must learn about their world only from the concrete—the "here and now."

5. *A social problem* Hearing-impaired children have difficulty developing appropriate behaviors towards other people. As toddlers they do not hear the tone of voice that indicates emotional state or signals the fact that they are about to transgress parental limits. At a later age they cannot have social rules explained to them. Even more importantly, they use manipulative and ritualistic behaviors as substitutes for language in their attempts to influence others.

6. *An emotional problem* Unable to satisfy their evolving needs with spoken language; unable to make sense of the seemingly precipitous and capricious reactions of parents and peers; constantly feeling acted upon rather than

acting upon others; hearing-impaired children become confused and angry and develop poor self-images.

7. *An educational problem* Children without language gain minimal benefit from educational experiences.

8. *An intellectual problem** Although it will be possible by suitable testing to demonstrate normal nonverbal intelligence, our subjects will be deficient in general knowledge and language competence—both of which are included in a broad definition of intelligence.

9. *A vocational problem* Lacking in verbal skills, general knowledge, academic training, and social skills, hearing-impaired children will reach adulthood with severely limited possibilities for gainful employment.

As if these secondary impairments were not enough, they are usually compounded by:

10. *Parental problems* The instinctive reactions of parents to a baby's failure to develop language is to withdraw language input and to reduce interaction. When they discover the true nature of the difficulties, they may well enter a state of denial and confusion which reduces their general effectiveness as parents and further undermines social and emotional development.

11. *Societal problems* The withdrawal of interaction by the parents will be repeated later by society at large.

It is small wonder that throughout most of recorded history the prospects for the young child with a severe, profound, or total hearing loss have been bleak. (See Figure 1–2.)

The case for intervention can be argued on ethical, moral, or humanistic grounds. If necessary, it can also be argued on economic grounds. The process I have just described produces adults who must be supported by others. If by intervention we can arrest this unfortunate chain of events, the same adults will become independent and contributing members of society.

○ INTERVENTION

The immediate goals of intervention are to reduce the primary impairment, to prevent the development of secondary problems, and to ensure that the evolving needs of the child and the family are met in spite of the hearing difficulty. The long term goal is an independent adult who is equipped to choose and to pursue his or her own road to personal fulfillment.

*Although intellectual function includes cognitive function, they are not the same thing. Through *cognition* individuals know the world in which they live. Through *intellect*, individuals use their world knowledge to solve problems—including those problems associated with acquiring and communicating information.

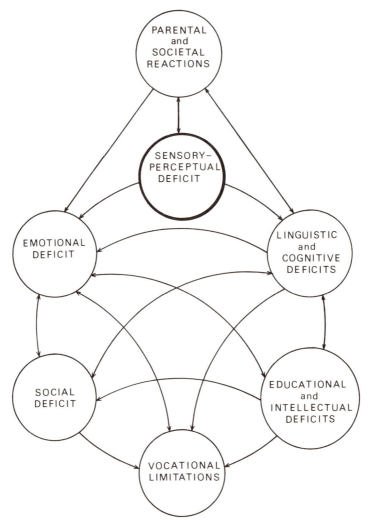

FIGURE 1–2 Without intervention, the consequences of hearing impairment in a young child are serious and far-reaching. The problems are accentuated by the instinctive reaction of parents and later, of society at large.

These goals can be addressed in four ways:

1. *Medical intervention* Drugs can be used in the treatment and prevention of hearing losses caused by middle ear infections. These losses are usually temporary but can become permanent. Note also that children who suffer recurring ear infections during the first few years of life may develop secondary auditory processing disorders despite successful medical intervention.

2. *Surgical intervention* Surgery is often used in the treatment of middle ear infections and in the correction of congenital abnormalities of the outer and middle ears. There have also been experiments on the surgical implantation of electrodes in the auditory nerve in an attempt to bypass defective inner ears, but the potential value of this procedure in the management of young hearing-impaired children is, at the time of writing, very much in doubt.

3. *Prosthetic intervention* The wearable electronic hearing aid, first developed in the 1930s, revolutionized the treatment of hearing loss. Countless numbers of children, who in earlier times would have been thought to be totally deaf, are now able to use hearing as the primary modality for acquiring spoken language skills. In consequence, they can function as hard-of-hearing individuals.

   Even those children for whom hearing aids provide only limited acoustic information learned better and faster if their auditory capacities are fully exploited by amplification. Hearing aids by no means restore normal hearing, but they can provide partial correction of most hearing losses.

   There have been many attempts to develop prosthetic devices, or sensory aids, that will help the hearing-impaired individual by converting sound into patterns of visual or tactile stimulation. Despite years of encouraging feasibility studies, such devices have not found general application.

4. *Habilitative intervention* Some hearing-impaired children stand to gain little or nothing from the three corrective measures just discussed, and even among those who do benefit, the majority will still have significant hearing impairments. Virtually all hearing-impaired children, therefore, require habilitative intervention. This form of intervention is essentially a preparation for life. It includes all interactions with the child, and all modifications of the physical and social environment that are designed to compensate for, or circumvent, primary impairments and to remediate, or prevent, secondary impairments. Although I shall refer to all four kinds of intervention, this book is concerned mainly with habilitation.

○ RATIONALE FOR EARLY INTERVENTION

It is easy to make a case for intervention, but why *early intervention*? Why can't we follow the practice of previous generations and wait until the child is old enough to enter school?

The reasons are several. First, early intervention permits us to focus on the *prevention* of secondary problems, rather than their *remediation*. This is an important point since it is in the secondary problems that the real difficulties of the hearing-impaired child lie. Lack of hearing is an inconvenience. Lack of communication with other human beings is a disaster. The child who reaches school age without having developed an effective language system is in serious jeopardy, and it may already be too late to undo the damage to social and emotional development.

The second reason relates to the concept of *critical age*. There is compelling evidence to suggest that children are neurologically ready to acquire basic perceptual skills and language skills during the first few years of life and that if advantage is not taken of this readiness, there may be irreversible neurological changes that interfere with learning at a later age. Many professionals object to the implication that it can become "too late" for hearing-impaired children to acquire language skills, but all agree that it is better to start as soon as the child is neurologically ready.

Directly related to the concept of readiness is that of *developmental synchrony*. Children progress along several parallel but interrelated tracks. There is, for example, motoric development, perceptual development, language development, social development, and so on. As needs appear in a given developmental area, they are often met by subskills developed in other areas. If, as a result of *developmental asynchrony*, particular subskills are not available, the child must find alternative ways of meeting certain needs, perhaps to the detriment of long term development. Consider, for example, children who cannot use language to meet their need to influence people. If, instead, they use tantrums or other manipulative behaviors, the foundations of social development, and, therefore, of language development, will be undermined.

By early intervention we, therefore, hope to

1. Maximize prevention.
2. Capitalize on critical age.
3. Preserve developmental synchrony.

The concept of early intervention is not new. It was advocated at least as early as 1680. Only since the 1940s, however, has it become accepted practice. Early intervention was made feasible by early identification, wearable hearing aids, improved knowledge, and changing professional attitudes. European educators took the lead in developing practical programs, to be followed some ten or twenty years later by their American colleagues. A major impetus was provided by the rubella epidemic of the early 1960s, which temporarily tripled, or quadrupled, the number of hearing-impaired infants. There were, however, several individuals and centers in the United States already committed to this work. Particular mention should be made of the pioneering efforts of the John Tracy Clinic, which was founded in 1943. Its correspondence course for the parents of hearing-impaired children has had international impact and was for many years a mainstay of early intervention.

○ RESULTS OF EARLY INTERVENTION

How successful is early intervention? After thirty or forty years of experience we might expect that this question would be easy to answer. Unfortunately, it is not. There are few norms for the development of young hearing-impaired children, so it is difficult to evaluate an individual child's progress in terms of the expected performance of children with the same etiology, degree of hearing loss, time of acquisition, intelligence, and cultural background. Ethical considerations make it almost impossible to carry out controlled research studies in which intervention is given to one group but withheld from another group, and retrospective studies are plagued by the effects of uncontrolled variables. To make matters worse, there is an unfortunate tendency on the part of educators to demonstrate the success of their programs by describing only their star students, leaving the impression that these students are typical. Such techniques serve only to confuse the objective observer and to discredit the programs in question.

In the absence of scientific data (and sometimes in spite of them), the best way to evaluate the success of early intervention programs is to listen to the opinions of experienced and open-minded educators who are familiar with the range of attainments typical of children with various types and degrees of hearing impairment. On the strength of such evidence it is clear that countless numbers of hearing-impaired children have had their life opportunities dramatically expanded by early intervention. This is particularly true of those children who have been transformed from *deaf* to *hard-of-hearing* by modern hearing aids and proper auditory management. Before the 1940s, such children accounted for at least 50 percent of the population in schools for the deaf. Today many of them acquire sufficient command of spoken language that they can enter school with normally hearing children at age five.

It must be acknowledged, however, that early intervention is not universally successful. Some children gain nothing, while others lose their "head start" after a few years of primary school. Some possible reasons for failure are as follows:

1. The parents, by virtue of personality, education, cultural background, or life circumstances, are unable to modify their behaviors in order to meet the child's special needs.

2. The child has perceptual, intellectual, symbolic, or other primary impairments in addition to the hearing impairment.

3. The particular method to which the child was exposed is incompatible with his or her needs. (An example of this would be the use of an exclusively auditory approach with a totally deaf child.)

4. The skills developed during early intervention are not sustained, capitalized on, and reinforced at the preprimary and primary levels.

5. The person providing habilitative intervention lacks the depth of experience and training needed to address the multiple needs of each child and family or to adapt to the differing needs of different children and their families.

The last of these problems provides the primary justification for the present text. As the concept of early intervention has become more widely accepted, and the techniques of early identification more effectively applied, the demand for services has increased. At the same time, improved neonatal care has resulted in the survival of increasing numbers of hearing-impaired children with additional neurological problems. Effective preparation of personnel requires assimilation of knowledge in several disciplines in addition to apprenticeship in successful early intervention programs. Unfortunately, the provision of training opportunities has not kept pace with demand. The result is that early intervention is frequently undertaken by persons with training in only one of the relevant disciplines, little or no apprenticeship, or apprenticeship in a method which is applicable to only one subgroup of the population of hearing-impaired children.

It is to these people that this book is primarily addressed. My purpose is to present a global view of the nature and management of hearing impairments in young children; to provide a logical, conceptual framework for developing intervention programs; and to offer suggestions for their implementation. Because there is only so much that can be accomplished by reading a single book, I have included a short bibliography at the end of most chapters. These reading suggestions should lead you to more detailed discussions of particular topics, supporting or conflicting viewpoints on various issues, or more practical advice on procedures. All of this reading should, of course, be combined with practice to be maximally effective. It is from the hearing-impaired children and their families that you will learn the most.

SUMMARY

Hearing is what happens when we detect and interpret minute disturbances in the air around us. In human beings, the sense of hearing plays a key role in the use and development of verbal language for communication. Hearing impairment has perceptual, communicative, speech, cognitive, social, emotional, educational, intellectual, and vocational consequences that are often compounded by the reactions of parents and society—hence the need for intervention.

Intervention can include medical, surgical, prosthetic, and habilitative components. The justification for early intervention is based on the concept of critical age and on the need to preserve developmental synchrony. Because of the complexity of the problem, the shortage of trained personnel, and the changing population of hearing-impaired children, early habilitative intervention can claim only partial success.

This book offers a conceptual framework and practical guidelines to help teachers address the general, special, and individual needs of hearing-impaired children and their families.

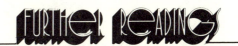

Excellent reviews of the history of education of the deaf, in general, and early intervention, in particular, will be found in Donald Moores' *Educating the Deaf* (Houghton Mifflin Co., Boston, 1978).

The results of early intervention—as they apply to language development—are reviewed by Stephen Quigley in *Pediatric Audiology,* edited by F. N. Martin (Prentice-Hall, Inc., Englewood Cliffs, N.J. 1978).

Other useful sources of information on the results of specific methods are Ciwa Griffiths' *Conquering Childhood Deafness* (Exposition Press, New York, 1967), Doreen Pollack's *Educational Audiology for the Limited Hearing Infant* (Chas. C Thomas, Springfield, Ill., 1970), and a paper by Daniel Ling and Muriel Milne entitled "The Development of Speech in Hearing-Impaired Children," in *Amplification in Education,* edited by F. H. Bess (A. G. Bell Association for the Deaf, Washington, D.C., 1981).

For information on medical, surgical, and prosthetic intervention, I refer you to Burton F. Jaffe's *Hearing Loss in Children* (University Park Press, Baltimore, Md., 1977) and particularly to Chapters 33 through 38 and Chapters 48 through 50.

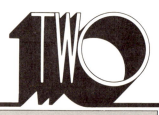

Normal hearing

In this chapter I review the processes by which we detect and interpret sound vibrations.

○ HEARING MECHANISMS

The hearing mechanism has three components: conductive, sensory, and neural, each of which has an essentially different function.

conductive component (see figure 2–1)

The conductive component consists of the outer and middle ears. Its function is to collect weak sound vibrations from the surrounding air and pass them to the fluids of the inner ear with as little loss of energy as possible. At the same time the conductive component helps protect the inner ear from the effects of loud noises and direct physical damage. It is fully developed at birth, though babies may have a conductive hearing loss for a few days after birth due to the presence of fluid in the middle ear cavity.

sensory component (see figure 2–2)

The sensory component of hearing is the *cochlea*. Its function is to separate the frequencies of complex sounds and to convert patterns of sound into patterns of nerve impulses. Directly attached to the cochlea are the organs of balance. Together, the hearing and balance organs make up the *inner ear*.

It is important to realize that the cochlea does not simply transform sound energy into neural energy. It is an encoding device that translates the language of sound into the language of the brain. The patterns generated by the cochlea provide the brain with *information about* sound. This information is rich and detailed. The cochlea is capable of differentiating over 100 levels of intensity between the thresholds of audibility and pain and over 1000 different values of frequency within the audible frequency range. The cochlea provides information on the time of arrival of high frequency sounds with an accuracy of better than one-tenth of one-thousandth of a

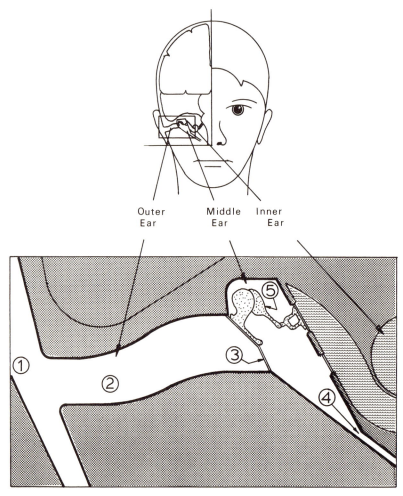

FIGURE 2-1 The conductive component of the hearing mechanism (simplified). The function of the conductive component is to transfer sound vibrations from the outside air to the fluids of the inner ear with as little loss of energy as possible. The auricle (1) collects sounds and directs them into the ear canal (2) along which they travel to the eardrum (3). The eustachian tube (4) allows air into, or out of, the middle ear space, thus maintaining the proper air pressure and allowing the eardrum to vibrate freely. The eardrum vibrates in step with the sound patterns, causing the ossicles (5) to vibrate. The ossicles are three small bones that form a bridge across the middle ear space and transfer the sound vibrations to the fluids of the inner ear.

second. It can also transmit information on the relative strengths of hundreds of simultaneously occurring tones.

The sensory component of hearing is fully developed at birth, but it takes many years for the brain to learn how to use all of the information provided by this remarkable organ.

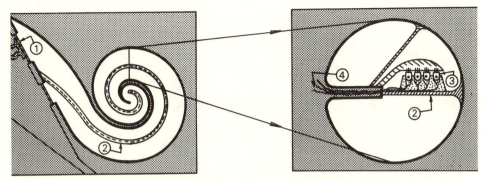

FIGURE 2–2 The sensory component of the hearing mechanism (simplified). A lengthwise section of the cochlea is shown on the left; a cross section on the right. The function of the cochlea is to convert patterns of sound into patterns of nerve impulses. Sound vibrations enter the cochlea at the round window membrane (1) and cause vibrations of the cochlear partition (2). The resulting stimulation of the hair cells (3) produces electrical impulses in the nerve fibers (4) leading to the brain.

neural component (see figure 2–3.)

The neural component of hearing consists of the auditory nerve and all those parts of the brain concerned with processing the information generated by the cochlea. Strictly speaking, it also includes the nerve fibers within the cochlea itself. Between the cochlea and the auditory cortex there are several processing centers, each containing thousands of nerve cells. These processing centers have complex interconnections involving both ascending and descending nerve fibers (that is, fibers carrying information from lower to higher levels in the brain and fibers carrying information the other way). Nerve cells communicate with each other at synapses. Essentially each cell decides whether or not to generate its own impulses by comparing the impulses it receives at facilitatory synapses with those it receives at inhibitory synapses. The net result of the thousands of decisions made within the processing centers constitutes auditory perception.

Unlike the conductive and sensory components, the neural component of hearing is neither fully developed nor fully functional at birth. During the first year of life, children lay down new neural connections and complete the myelinization of nerve fibers in order to speed up the transmission of impulses; and during the first few years of life they develop auditory perception, that is, they learn how to hear.

site of lesion tests

In clinical hearing evaluations a major goal is to find out which part of the hearing mechanism is damaged. For example, a comparison of air conduction sensitivity and bone conduction sensitivity may identify dis-

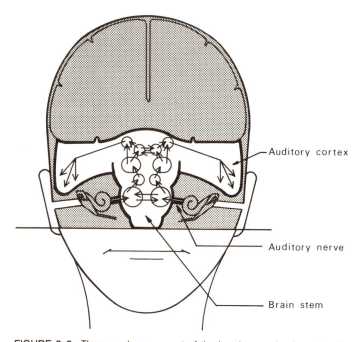

FIGURE 2–3 The neural component of the hearing mechanism (simplified). Patterns of nerve impulses generated by the cochlea pass along the auditory nerve to the brain stem where they are processed in various centers. Information from these centers eventually reaches the auditory cortex. Note that each side of the brain receives information from both right and left ears. Note also that whereas this diagram suggests that information passes in only one direction, from cochlea to cortex, auditory processing also involves the transfer of information in the opposite direction.

orders of the conductive component; *tympanometry*—a procedure in which we assess the effects of changing air pressure in the ear canal on the sound reflected from the eardrum—may provide clues about the nature of conductive disorders; investigation of speech discrimination and the perception of loudness may identify disorders in the cochlea; and measures of the ability to integrate and/or separate information presented to the two ears may reveal disorders of the neural component.

○ AUDITORY PERCEPTION

It can be helpful to think of perception as asking questions about objects and events in our environment and answering those questions using evidence provided by our sense organs. In auditory perception we are concerned mainly with events, since it is events that involve the movements that generate sound.

Auditory perception involves several subprocesses.

ity. You should note, however, that physiological techniques such as ctrocochleography or evoked response audiometry provide direct esti- ates of capacity.

discrimination

Related to the process of detection is that of discrimination. This process involves asking and answering the question, "Was this sound differ- ent from that sound?"

Discrimination capacity is determined entirely by the cochlea. It cannot be improved by either amplification or training. *Discrimination performance* is determined by the neural mechanism of hearing. It can be improved by training but only up to the limits set by discrimination capacity. In most people, discrimination performance is considerably poorer than discrimina- tion capacity. That is to say, they are capable of making much finer distinc- tions than they actually use for the identification and recognition of sound patterns.

Neonates show evidence of discrimination performance by responding differently to different sounds and by habituating to repeated sounds. Be- cause of their limited response repertoire, however, we are unable to deter- mine the limits of their discrimination capacity.

Techniques for the measurement of discrimination capacity have been developed for research purposes, but they are not applied in standard clinical hearing tests. Instead we usually infer discrimination performance from the results of word recognition tests.

sensation

When we ask the question, "What was the sound like?" the answer is experienced as an auditory sensation. This sensation can have many dimensions. For example,

loudness dependent mainly on sound intensity

tonicity dependent on periodicity of the sound waveform

pitch dependent mainly on fundamental frequency

quality dependent on time envelope and spectrum

harmony dependent on ratios of simultaneous fundamental frequencies

melody dependent on ratios of sequential fundamental frequencies, and so on.

This list is actually open-ended. With increasing experience of more and more complex sounds, our ability to respond to the structure of sound

attention

We must first decide whether to ask questions an
questions to ask. The resulting processes of arousal, listening,
distraction are usually discussed under the heading of attent
these processes are believed to be the responsibility of that par
called the *reticular formation.* Others may involve the frontal lo

Babies demonstrate primitive arousal and listening behaviors
before, birth and refine these skills during the first few years of
lems of auditory attention result from neurological damage or se
privation. Standard clinical testing does not include assessmen
function.

detection

Auditory detection is the process of asking and answering the
tion, "Was there a sound?" If enough acoustic energy reaches the co
to produce a significant change in the neural activity of the auditory pro
ing centers, we detect the *sound* and we experience the sensation of *so*
(Note that the word sound is used to refer both to the physical vibrati
of the air and to the sensations produced by those vibrations. Failure
appreciate this double use leads people into futile arguments about wheth
a sound exists when no one hears it.)

Except in cases of extensive neural damage, the *detection capacity* of the
hearing mechanism is determined by the integrity of conductive and sensory
mechanisms. Detection capacity can be improved prosthetically by amplification but not by training. *Detection performance,* on the other hand, is determined by the neural mechanism. Detection performance can be improved
by training but only up to the limits of detection capacity. When we measure
the threshold of hearing, we are measuring detection performance. In most
cases there is little difference between capacity and performance, but among
young, sensorially deprived or neurologically impaired children, there can
be large discrepancies. With maturation, training, or both, the detection
performance of such children often improves, sometimes leading to the
mistaken conclusion that their detection capacity has increased (that is, that
their hearing loss has diminished).

In spite of a limited response repertoire, it has been demonstrated that
the detection capacity of neonates is normal. This implies that babies are
able to hear the sounds of their mother's circulatory and digestive systems
for some time before birth. What is frequently overlooked is that they have
also been able to hear their mothers' speech, an experience that may contribute to social and communicative development in the young child.

Measurement of *detection performance* constitutes the major portion of
standard hearing evaluations, the results being used to infer detection ca-

patterns is unlimited. Of particular importance to human development is the awareness of those structures peculiar to human speech.

Since auditory sensations are internal to the perceiver, we have no way of knowing how they are experienced by a neonate or how they are affected by sensory and neural hearing impairments. Even when an individual has a unilateral sensory impairment, his or her ability to describe the sound sensations evoked by the defective ear is limited by lack of a shared vocabulary.

localization

Sound localization requires asking and answering the question, "Where did the sound originate?"

Sound provides a rich source of information about the direction and distance of the events that produce it and about the direction and distance of the surfaces that reflect it. Hearing, therefore, plays an important role in the development of space perception and relieves us of the necessity for constant visual scanning. Auditory localization skills also contribute to auditory attentional processes. Localization capacity is determined by both the sensory and neural mechanisms of hearing and requires the ability to interpret subtle differences in the intensity, spectra, and times of arrival of sounds reaching the two ears.

Even at a few weeks of age, babies demonstrate primitive localization performance by searching for the source of a sound and turning their heads in its general direction. By nine months they immediately turn to focus on the source—indicating that they can answer the question, "Where did the sound originate?" even before they know what made the sound. Sound localization skills are not usually assessed in clinical hearing evaluations.

recognition

Auditory recognition requires asking and answering the question, "What made the sound?" The answer is an object or an event. Before children can answer this question, they must have begun to organize their sensory experiences into a world of objects and events, otherwise they have no answers to give. This means that the development of auditory recognition skills is just one aspect of general perceptual development.

The skills of auditory recognition are entirely learned. They appear in the young baby at about three months of age and develop very rapidly in the first two years of life. After this they continue to develop indefinitely, though more slowly.

Although the process of recognition takes place in the neural mechanism, it cannot occur unless sound patterns are detected. Nor can it occur if the cochlea lacks the ability to differentiate among sounds that are produced by different events. You should note, however, that the auditory information provided by the cochlea is only one of the sources of information on which recognition is based. We also have evidence from other sensory inputs and from situational and temporal contexts.

Standard clinical testing does include measurement of auditory recognition performance, but this is usually restricted to word recognition.

comprehension

The ultimate goal of auditory perception in humans is not to determine whether a sound was present, where it came from, or what made it, but to answer the question, "Why was the sound made?"

Recognition is a prerequisite for comprehension, but whereas recognition is a backward-looking process in which the present stimulus is evaluated in terms of past experience, comprehension is a forward-looking process in which our knowledge of the rules and relationships governing the world is used to infer the *meaning* of a particular sound's occurrence at a particular time and in a particular place.

One could argue that we do not determine the significance of the sound itself but of the event which caused it and that comprehension is a general cognitive process that is independent of a specific modality. Nevertheless, there are certain events that are perceived almost exclusively through hearing, and there are individuals who appear to have difficulty with comprehension only when events are perceived through hearing. The concept of auditory comprehension may therefore be a useful one.

Comprehension is a neural process and is entirely dependent on learning. Its appearance in young children must await the beginnings of conceptual development between twelve and eighteen months of age. Standard clinical tests of hearing do not include an evaluation of auditory comprehension.

auditory memory

If auditory perception is to be successful, we must retain auditory images. For example

We need to retain one part of an auditory pattern while waiting for the next part.

We need to retain the complete auditory image while making decisions about its attributes, its nature, or its significance.

We need to retain one auditory image if we are to differentiate it from another.

We need to retain auditory images for long periods of time if we are to develop auditory recognition skills.

It is probable that many different kinds of memory are involved in these activities, but we tend to discuss them under one heading—*auditory memory*. In keeping with the model of auditory perception I have presented so far, we might define this skill as remembering the answers to questions about sound patterns.

Auditory memory is fundamental to the development and application of auditory perception. We know that neonates exhibit performance in this area by virtue of their alerting and habituation behaviors. We have very little understanding of the process, however, and few tools with which to measure performance in a clinical setting.

○ SPEECH PERCEPTION

Among the many events that we perceive by means of hearing, the events of speech form a special class. They are special for two reasons. First, they are made by people and therefore are important to social development and interaction. Secondly, they are used to encode linguistic structures which are themselves an encoding of conceptually organized thought.

The events of speech can be perceived, at least partially, by means of the senses of vision and touch. They are intended, however, for perception by means of the sense of hearing, and it is only through this modality that full perception is possible.

The intensity of conversational speech fluctuates rapidly within the range 30 dB to 60 dB above the threshold of normal hearing. *Detection* of speech is therefore possible for persons whose hearing sensitivity is within 60 dB of normal, though full audibility requires sensitivity within 30 dB of normal.

The acoustic speech code is relatively crude compared with the *discrimination* capacity of normal ears. In fact, persons with sensory hearing losses up to 60 dB have sufficient capacity to differentiate all the linguistically significant speech events.

Speech *recognition* operates at several possible levels. When we ask, "What made the sound?" we can do so in terms of

> *speech movements* What movements produced that sound pattern? (This we can answer because we are ourselves generators of speech and therefore know the association between speech sound and speech movement).
>
> *sex* Is it a male or a female speaker?
>
> *age* Is it a child or an adult, and so on?
>
> *emotional state* Is the person happy, angry, scared, and so on?
>
> *health* Does the person have a cold, laryngitis, and so on?
>
> *national origin* Is it an American, a Russian, and so on?

regional origin Is it a southerner, a midwesterner, and so on?

syntactic boundaries Is that the end of a sentence, and so on?

emphasis and stress Is that an important word or syllable, and so on?

vocabulary What word does that sound pattern represent?

phonology What speech sound does that sound pattern represent?

subphonemic features Was that sound voiced or unvoiced, and so on?

Similarly, speech *comprehension* operates at several levels. When we ask, "Why was the sound made?" our answer may be the meaning of a sentence, or we may ask about hidden meanings, symbolism, or motivation. Comprehending a question such as, "Would you like to come up to my room for a drink?" for example, requires more than linguistic competence.

Assessment of speech perception ability and performance in the hearing clinic is usually limited to measures of speech detection and the recognition of words.

SUMMARY

The hearing mechanism has three components: conductive, sensory, and neural. The conductive component transfers energy. The sensory component converts sound patterns into neural patterns. The neural component interprets neural patterns.

The function of the neural component may be thought of as asking and answering questions about the sound patterns and the information those patterns contain. This process we call auditory perception. The questions we ask concern the presence and characteristics of the sound, the position and nature of its source, and the reason for its existence. Attention and short term memory are important subskills.

Speech perception is a special skill which is primarily auditory but may also employ vision and touch. The questions to be asked and answered concern the units of a language code, the thoughts conveyed by a speaker, and the purpose of the speaker in expressing those thoughts.

The conductive and sensory components of hearing are fully developed and functional at, or soon after, birth. The neural component is not. Both physical maturation and learning are required for the full development of auditory perceptual skills.

Tests of hearing are concerned mainly with finding out which parts of the mechanism are damaged, measuring detection ability, and measuring word recognition performance. Many aspects of auditory perception are ignored in clinical evaluation. Some of these aspects are of central importance to the process we call *hearing*.

FURTHER READINGS

    A very readable description of the normal hearing mechanism may be found in Lawrence Deutsch and Alan Richards' *Elementary Hearing Science* (University Park Press, Baltimore, Md., 1979). For more in-depth reading, I suggest *Pediatric Audiology,* edited by F. N. Martin (Prentice-Hall, Inc., Englewood Cliffs, New Jersey, 1978), and Jerry Northern and Marion Downs' *Hearing in Children,* second edition (Williams & Wilkins, Baltimore, Md., 1978). These two texts also contain good descriptions of the development of auditory behavior in children.

    The general topic of auditory perception is not well treated in the literature, but a very exhaustive account of auditory skills in newborns is presented by Rita Eisenberg in *Auditory Competence in Early Life* (University Park Press, Baltimore, Md., 1976).

    Descriptions and discussions of speech perception abound in the literature, but none is entirely comprehensive. I suggest you start with Derek Sanders' book *Auditory Perception of Speech* (Prentice-Hall, Inc., Englewood Cliffs, N.J., 1977) and the chapters by Daniel Ling and Arthur Boothroyd in *Auditory Management of Hearing Impaired Children,* edited by M. Ross and T. G. Giolas (University Park Press, Baltimore, Md., 1978). These will provide you with extensive references if you wish to study the topic further.

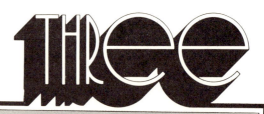

THREE

Child development
and normal hearing

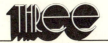

No one should attempt to intervene in the development of young hearing-impaired children without a thorough understanding of normal development and the role that hearing plays in this process. In this chapter I review those aspects of development which are dependent, directly or indirectly, on hearing. They are speech development, cognitive and language development, and social and emotional development.

○ THE DEVELOPMENTAL PROCESS

Before discussing specific areas of development, there are some aspects of the process itself that need to be mentioned.

nature and nurture

Newborn babies are equipped with a remarkable array of reflexes, drives, capacities, and predispositions, and they grow in an environment of objects, people, and events which affect them. The course of development is determined both by the child's intrinsic characteristics and by environmental influences. More precisely, it is determined by the interplay between the two.

Our present concern is with children who are deficient in a very basic capacity—that of hearing. We hope to minimize the effects of this instrinsic shortcoming by suitable modifications of the environment.

parallel and sequential development

Young children develop in several areas at the same time. For example, they develop motorically, socially, intellectually, and linguistically. Within each area they must follow a predetermined developmental sequence. That is to say, they must progress from one stage to the next in a certain order. The time of transition to a new developmental stage is determined by three things: intrinsic drives and needs, environmental demands, and possession of the necessary *readiness* skills. In many instances these skills originate in other developmental areas than the one in which they are expressed. For example, children cannot learn to talk in sentences until they have the necessary cognitive skills and motor skills. Thus, although the

25

developmental areas are different, they are by no means independent. This fact should be kept in mind when we artifically separate specific areas for discussion.

developmental synchrony

The normal child in a normal environment is characterized by developmental synchrony. That is to say, as intrinsic needs emerge, the necessary readiness skills and environmental conditions are available. He or she thus proceeds smoothly from one stage of development to the next. Serious deficiencies of basic capacities or of environmental circumstances may lead to developmental asynchrony. That is to say, intrinsic needs emerge before the child has the necessary readiness skills or in the absence of the proper input from the environment. If this problem is not resolved, the needs may be satisfied in inappropriate ways and development impaired. It is important to realize that a child who has all the basic capacities, but is developing slowly in one area, may become seriously handicapped simply because of developmental asynchrony.

critical age

Closely related to the foregoing discussion is the concept of critical age. The greater the length of time that elapses between the emergence of a developmental need and the establishment of the necessary subskills and environmental conditions, the more difficult it becomes for development to follow its proper course. It is not clear whether this is because of changes in neurological receptivity or because of the secondary consequences of developmental asynchrony. Most probably, both factors are important.

Piaget

The contribution of Jean Piaget to the subject of child development has been considerable. Much of the standard terminology in this field is derived from his work, and while the details of his theories may be the subject of debate, their basic framework is widely accepted. Perhaps his most significant contribution has been to describe development from the child's perspective. Piaget has shown us the child, not as an imperfect adult, but as a cognitively active individual who is complete at each developmental stage. Although his studies were mostly carried out with normal children, I believe their results have wide applicability to handicapped children, including those with impaired hearing. In the descriptions that follow I draw heavily on Piaget's theories of development.

○ SPEECH DEVELOPMENT

Speech is a system of movements that generate sounds. It provides a medium by which human beings can exchange linguistically coded thoughts. Speech competence develops spontaneously during the first four or five years of life and is virtually complete at the end of this time. Among the prerequisites are

adequate exposure to the speech of others

the ability to hear and explore self-generated speech sounds

adequate cognitive and linguistic development

the opportunity to interact with one or more persons who already use speech as a medium for communication

association of speech sounds and speech movements

Fundamental to normal speech development is the establishment of an intimate association between the sounds of speech and the movements that generate them. The two must become inseparably connected in the child's brain, like two sides of the same coin. Since they hear every sound they make, normally hearing children have ample opportunity to establish this association—beginning with the birth cry and continuing through reflexive vocalization, babbling, imitation, and communication.

reflexive vocalization

For the first few weeks of life, babies are passive receivers of the sounds they make. They hear their own cries, gurgles, coughs, and sneezes but have no voluntary control over the existence or form of these noises. Nevertheless, this is an important stage since the connections between speech sounds and speech movements are being established. At the same time, babies are passive receivers of speech sounds from others. This also is important since the patterns of their native language are being imprinted in their brains and in many cases are becoming associated with the satisfaction of needs.

purposeful vocalization

By two or three months of age babies discover that they can control the existence of their own speech sounds, just as they can control the accessibility of their hands. They are engaged in what Piaget calls a *primary circular reaction.* That is to say, they deliberately and directly generate their own sensory stimuli.

exploration and imitation

The next stage of development occurs when babies begin to experiment with the form of the sounds they can make. They start to coo, sing, and experiment with simple syllables. They are still learning to associate sound and movement, but they are also learning to control them both.

At about six months of age these explorations become selective. Babies begin to spend more time generating the kinds of sound patterns they have been hearing from the people around them. They begin to imitate both the rhythmic, melodic, and phonetic features of their native language.

These exploratory activities are noticed by the babies' parents, who reinforce them by further imitation. They "babble" back. This sets the stage for what Piaget calls *secondary circular reaction.* Not only do children generate their own babbling, but they cause other people to make the same sounds. They can also cause other people to appear by purposeful vocalization—a great improvement on the earlier use of reflexive vocalizations brought on by discomfort.

communication

As their imitative skills improve, young children of fourteen or fifteen months of age begin to produce whole words. They have already learned, in their interactions with other people, that these words are associated with particular objects or events, and they have developed a fairly advanced understanding of the material world in which they live. They can now produce *tertiary circular reactions,* in which their vocal outputs cause other people to perform certain acts or satisfy certain needs. They are using speech for communication. From this point on, the major development in speech competence will be a refinement of articulation and a shift away from auditory control to proprioceptive and kinesthetic control.

proprioceptive and kinesthetic control

As the young child learns to associate the sounds and movements of speech, he or she also experiences the *feel* of speech. This tactile feedback may, in fact, play an important role in the transition from reflexive vocalization to purposeful vocalization. Throughout the process of exploration and imitation and the beginnings of communication, however, it is not the feel of speech that is important but the *sound* of speech. Development and control are being directed by the child's hearing.

Hearing will continue to play the primary role in ensuring the correct production of loudness, voice quality, and pitch throughout life. This is not so for rhythm and articulation, however. Between their second and fourth birthdays, children begin paying less attention to the sounds of their own speech and rely more on their memory of how speech should feel. As they get older, it becomes more and more difficult for children to acquire new articulation skills through hearing, and after puberty it is almost impossible.

○ COGNITIVE AND LINGUISTIC DEVELOPMENT

There are several theories of the nature of language, the process of language acquisition, and the relationship between language and thought. The following discussion is based on the belief that language is an essential component of human cognitive function and its acquisition an inevitable outcome of cognitive development in a child who interacts with language users.

nature of cognition and language

Cognition is the process of knowing the world in which we exist. Our only access to this world is through neural patterns that are generated by our sense organs in response to physical stimulation. We are driven to explain these patterns, and in the process we develop an internal description of reality (or to use Piaget's term, a *schema*). It is as though we construct a personal model of the world. An appreciation of the concept of an internal, personal model of reality is, I believe, central to an understanding of human development. For the purposes of the present text I shall refer to this as a *world model*.

Language consists of two things: a set of symbols by which individuals can refer to components of their world models and a set of rules for selecting, modifying, and arranging these symbols for the purpose of conveying ideas between human beings.

The two processes—cognition and language—are interdependent. Adequate cognitive development is a prerequisite for language development and once developed, language becomes a powerful tool for promoting further cognitive development. Without the tool of language, an individual's cognitive development must remain at a primitive, concrete level. Language frees people from the limitations of the immediate and the familiar. Language provides access to a world which can extend backwards and forwards in time and outward in space. Language gives the individual access to the accumulated experience of human society.

mechanisms of cognitive development

Cognitive development involves two processes: assimilation and accommodation. *Assimilation* is the accumulation of sensory experience and its incorporation into an existing world model. Assimilation requires attention, one or more functional sensory systems, and memory. *Accommodation* is the reorganization of the world model to allow for sensory experiences that by virtue of their nature or quantity are incompatible with the existing model. It is important to realize that this model is always complete, but at the same time never finished. The young child's world model *is* reality as he or she knows it. It may seem immature in comparison with our own, just as our own may seem immature in twenty or thirty years' time.

An important aid to cognitive development is *exploration,* or the generation of circular reactions. By voluntary motor acts, individuals can partially control their own sensory experience and at the same time, test their world model. So important is this process during the first two years of life that Piaget refers to this time as the *sensorimotor* stage of development. (See Figure 3–1).

It is important to realize that the world model is improved by both assimilation and accommodation. One leads to greater complexity, the other, through hierarchial reorganization, to greater simplicity. These opposing trends continue throughout life, beginning with the (relative) innocence of early childhood and progressing through the (relative) wisdom of old age.

When individuals undertake a major reorganization of their world models, they are observed to move into a new developmental stage. The timing of the transitions appears to depend partly on biological maturation and partly on the pressures of accumulated experience. I shall defer discussion of the developmental timetable until we have dealt with the mechanisms of language development.

mechanisms of language development

There are many prerequisites for the spontaneous development of language in young children. Among them are the following:

1. A world model that is organized into a system of discrete categories.
2. The ability to refer to these categories by symbols.
3. The opportunity to engage in communicative interactions with other people.
4. The sensory mechanism by which other people's language symbols can be perceived.
5. The sensorimotor mechanisms by which these same symbols can be generated.

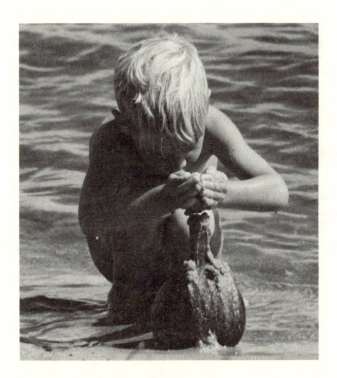

FIGURE 3-1 The developing child interacts with the world of "things" through motoric exploration. In the process he acquires information that can be incorporated into an expanding world model thus promoting cognitive growth.

Our major concern in the present text is obviously with the last two requirements which, under normal circumstances, are met by the hearing and speech mechanisms.

Exploration is as important to language development as it is to cognitive development. Young children discover the strengths and limitations of their language by trying it out on other people. They become aware of the need for improvement because they fail to communicate the intended idea or because they hear their utterances rephrased in a more correct form, that is, one which corresponds with the language rules of the society in which they live (see Figure 3-2).

Language development occurs in several areas. For example,

1. *Vocabulary* expansion of the symbol set.

2. *Semantics* refinement of the conceptual categories to which the symbols refer.

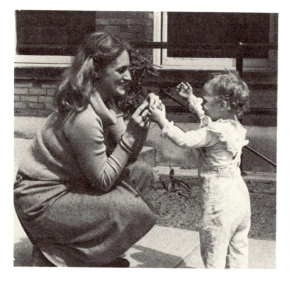

FIGURE 3–2 The developing child interacts with the world of people through both non-verbal and verbal dialogue. In the process she acquires information that can be incorporated into an expanding world model as well as information that can be incorporated into a language system. This interaction promotes social, emotional, cognitive, and linguistic growth.

3. *Syntax* expansion of the rules for selecting, modifying, and combining symbols.

4. *Pragmatics* expansion of the uses of language to include such things as control, requesting information, narration, and persuasion.

Linguists refer to these areas under the headings of content, form, and use.

Language development, like cognitive development, progresses through several stages. Because of their interrelationship, however, the two are discussed together.

developmental stages

In the first stage of cognitive-linguistic development, which begins at, or even before, birth, children are passive receivers of sensory impressions, some of which are generated by their own movements. As they retain and accumulate these impressions, they show increasing awareness of qualities, patterns, similarities, differences, and correspondences. At the very outset, babies habituate to a repeated stimulus and show preferences for certain stimulus patterns and within a few months they can be conditioned. The linguistic significance of this stage is considerable. In it children learn to associate the sounds of speech with other aspects of human contact; they become familiar with the sound patterns of their native language, and they begin to associate movements of their own speech apparatus with the resulting sounds.

The second stage begins at about three or four months. It is characterized by rapid perceptual development, motor development, and perceptual-motor exploration. Essentially, children learn that they can explain an otherwise confusing array of sensory impressions if they assume that these come from a concrete world of permanent objects and predictable events. Children use their developing motor skills to manipulate objects, and they learn more about how the objects feel, how they taste, how they look, and how they sound. They also learn the associations between these sensory modalities as they crawl, climb, and eventually walk around their environment, continually exploring and learning.

Several aspects of this stage have a bearing on language. The conscious mastery of motor skills permits exploration of the sounds that can be made with the speech mechanism. As children explore they begin to imitate the sound patterns they hear from other people. They discover that the sounds of speech are an effective way of manipulating people, and their physical explorations bring them into contact with the limits of acceptable behavior —the social consequences of which become associated with recognizable speech patterns.

But the most significant aspect of this stage of development is that the child's world model has been organized on a categorical basis. Whereas sensory impressions cover a broad continuum, with infinite possibilities for variation, their perceptual organization places them into a finite number of categories. The child can look at an object and place it into the correct category, that is, recognize it, despite variations of distance, orientation, and lighting, all of which change the image reaching his or her eye. Of particular importance is that fact that the child learns to recognize an object when only a part of it is visible or when shown a picture of it.

It should also be realized that the categories in this perceptual model have several sensory dimensions, any one of which can be used for recognition. *Mommy,* for example, can be recognized from her appearance, or the sound of her voice, or her feel, or her smell. What is more to the point, she can be *recognized* on the basis of sound patterns which have become associated with other ways of experiencing her—such as the spoken word *Mommy.* In other words, verbal labels can become a means of access to perceptual categories—they can become symbols for those categories.

With increasing mastery of speech skills, imitations are expanded to include words and commonly used phrases. This permits the child to use spoken utterances symbolically to convey to others that a particular perceptual category is uppermost in his or her consciousness.

Thus, by the time children reach one and a half or two years of age, they have a well-developed internal model of their world as a system of objects and events, many of which are associated with verbal labels, or symbols. Their receptive language skills consist of the ability to respond appropriately to sentences by recognizing one or more words and interpreting them in the light of the immediate situation. Their expressive language skills consist of the ability to make their thoughts and wishes known by the use of single words or commonly used phrases—again with the support of information from the immediate situation. They are also adept at using intonational patterns of speech for both receptive and expressive purposes.

At around two years of age, the child moves into a third developmental stage as his or her world model becomes too large and complicated to be handled on a purely perceptual level. There are too many objects and too many events, and another level of organization is required. New categories are therefore created on the basis of properties, functions, and relationships that are abstracted from concrete experience. These may be called conceptual categories. They do not contain real objects and events but consist of all possible examples of classes of objects and events. Categories are also created for such things as sensory and physical qualities, spatial and temporal relationships, and emotional states. The boundaries of these categories are no longer determined by the limitations of the physical world but by the rules which are assumed to govern it.

The new categories can still be accessed by verbal labels; however, the labels are used in a new way. As a perceptual label, the word *Mother* relates to a particular person and all the experiences with which she is associated. But as a conceptual label, it can refer to a large class of people, or animals, or even inanimate objects and abstract ideas, all of which share certain attributes. Think, for example, of the progression of the use of the word *Mother* in the following:

> *Mother* = my primary care giver.
>
> *Julie's mother* = the person who bears the same relationship to Julie as my mother bears to me.
>
> *The kitty's mother* = the animal that bears the same relationship to the kitten as mothers bear to children.
>
> *Mother Earth* = the land in terms of its relationship to the living creatures it produces and nurtures.
>
> *Necessity is the mother of invention* = two abstract concepts having a cause-effect relationship similar to that between mother and child.

Although the child's world model is now reorganized at a conceptual level, the verbal messages he or she receives and generates must still refer to the concrete world. But this creates a problem. How can symbols that stand for general conceptual categories be used to refer to specific objects and events? The answer is to be found in the sentence. This is a combination of two or more verbal labels which, by virtue of modifications of form and sequence, can become specific and can convey information about relationships. The sentence provides a sort of cross referencing system. When the two general labels *Father* and *my* are combined into *my father* a particular object is defined just as a point on a map is defined by two coordinates. Less precision is attained by adding the article "a" to "cake," but something very definite has been said about quantity. When "my father" and "a cake" appear in a sentence, there are several possible events that might connect the two. If we take the general label "make" and modify it appropriately, we become specific about the event, and we also limit the time frame for its occurrence—as in "My father made a cake." If more temporal precision is required, we can add other general labels such as "yesterday."

Children have learned the labels for perceptual categories by interacting with people who already use them. They must now learn the rules for generating sentences in the same way. Every sentence they hear, providing it relates to objects and events within their experience, is a potential source of information about grammatical rules. As children formulate rules and attempt to apply them, their successes and failures provide further information. If their messages are understood in spite of structural errors, they may hear their sentences rephrased by the people with whom they are talking.

Between the ages of two and five years, children develop an impressive conceptual model of the world, and they learn labels for a large number of conceptual categories. This set of labels is what linguists call a *lexicon*. Children also develop almost complete mastery of the rules for selecting, modifying, and sequencing those labels to make and understand sentences expressing relationships among two or more conceptual categories. This system of rules is what linguists call a *grammar*.

The fourth stage of development begins at four or five years of age, when the child has attained sufficient mastery of language for it to become independent of the concrete world. Conceptual development can now progress partly through purely verbal interactions with other people, either directly or by means of the printed word. Once children reach this stage, they can be "taught" in a formal educational setting. They have graduated from the "preschool" category and therefore from our immediate concern.

summary of development

To summarize, young children pass through four stages of cognitive development. In the first, they learn what their sense organs tell them about physical stimuli; in the second, they learn what physical stimuli tell them about the physical world; in the third, they learn what the physical world tells them about the rules by which it is governed; in the fourth, they use language as a supplement to the physical world.

Language development occurs at each stage. In the first stage, children gain familiarity with the sound patterns of their native language and learn to associate speech sounds and speech movements; in the second stage, they learn to use words as symbols for perceptual categories and as a means of influencing people; in the third stage, they begin to use words as symbols for conceptual categories and to generate sentences expressing relationships; in the fourth stage, their competence with language has reached the point where it can, if necessary, influence learning independently of experience.

I should stress that the transition of a child from one stage to the next does not involve the abandonment of earlier skills, or earlier learning styles, but rather the overlaying of new ones. It is as though there are several developmental tracks, each beginning at a different age but continuing throughout life. We need never stop developing sensory skills, perceptual skills, motor skills, conceptual skills, or language skills.

significance of dialogue

You, as the reader of this book, are engaged in activities characteristic of the fourth developmental stage. You are trying to learn something about the rules governing the physical world, through the medium of language. You are formulating new concepts and identifying them with verbal labels. Unfortunately, the labels I am offering are not entirely new to you. They are already used to identify concepts that may differ significantly from the ones presented here. Since we cannot interact, we are deprived of one of the most basic techniques by which human beings align their conceptual models and symbol systems—dialogue.

Dialogue, or conversation, is essential to the development of verbal language skills. It is an activity in which two people alternate in the roles of sender and receiver. They must also alternate in the roles of actor and reactor—a conversation does not occur if one person asks questions and the other simply answers them. Observations of mother-infant interactions indicate that the basic rules of conversation are established at a very early age. During the first two or three months, the mother plays both roles, the baby being a passive listener. But as soon as social smiling begins, mothers start to take their cues from their babies, replying to babies' smiles, their gazes, and later their gestures as though each were a sentence. It is probable that this early *preconversational* interaction is necessary for later language development. Once toddlers are able to generate full sentences, their capacity for conversation seems limitless. It may seem that children are gaining a lot of information during conversation, but in fact its primary purpose is the learning of language rules and the alignment of their verbal symbol systems with that of the society into which they were born. If habilitative intervention with the hearing-impaired child is to be effective, some way must be found of establishing preconversational and true conversational interactions.

thinking

So far I have said nothing about thinking or about the relationship between thinking and language. It is my belief that these are not two separate activities but two manifestations of the same activity and that both are dependent on the existence of a conceptually organized world model. When we perform internal operations on that model, we are thinking. When we externalize those operations, we are seen to be engaged in language activity. The basic problem for any language is that the external symbols are bound by constraints of space and time whereas the internal manipulations are not. It is the wide range of choices for mapping thought processes on to a system of physical symbols which accounts for the variety among human languages.

○ SOCIAL AND EMOTIONAL DEVELOPMENT

Social and emotional function may be defined as follows: An individual's perception of, and interaction with, self and others. Emotional development is obviously concerned mainly with *self* and social development with *others,* but the two are interdependent. Adequate emotional development requires adequate social development and vice versa.

Hearing plays a significant, but not essential, role in the early stages of emotional and social development, and language plays a significant *and* essential role in the later stages. Hence the inclusion of this topic in the present chapter.

cognitive aspects

Healthy social and emotional development depends initially on normal cognitive development. As babies begin to construct a world model, the first thing they must do is to establish a category for *self.* More precisely, they must divide their world model into two parts—*self* and *not self.* The first evidence of this emerges at about three months of age. Almost immediately, the category for *not self* is divided into two parts—*people* and *not people.* This process is aided by the baby's predisposition to attend auditorily to speechlike sounds and visually to facelike shapes. This is also the age at which the baby begins to smile at people—an activity which is rewarding to the people (despite its indiscriminate application) and is therefore reinforced.

Much has been written of the relationship that develops between mother and child, and any attempt to stress the significance of this relationship courts understatement. In a sense the child's mother fills the category of *people* when it is first established. By about four months of age, however, preference is shown for the real mother, implying that "people" has been subdivided into *mother* and *other people.* This occurrence is gratifying to the mother, who reinforces it by her reaction and thus helps to establish the mother-child bond.

At about eight months of age the category *other people* is further divided into *familiar people* and *strangers,* as evidenced by the child's growing wariness of people outside the nuclear family.

Further evidence of the interactions between cognitive and social and emotional development appear at about ten months when children begin to use people as a resource, and thirteen months when they demonstrate pride in their own achievements.

auditory aspects

Hearing is one of the modalities through which young babies discover themselves and other people, and it therefore contributes to the foundation of social and emotional development. Later, hearing provides information about the approach or the presence of other people even when they are not seen. It also serves to convey information about the emotional state of other people through intonation and tone of voice. There is no evidence, however, to indicate that hearing is indispensable in the early establishment of appropriate social and emotional function.

speech aspects

The baby's early efforts at purposeful and communicative vocalization have a profound effect on his or her parents and serve as reinforcers and triggers of certain essential behaviors on their part. In this connection we must remember that the baby does not develop in a static environment, but influences other people just as these other people influence the baby. In fact, everything that I said earlier about developmental synchrony and critical ages can be applied equally well to the development of the mother-child unit and later of the family-child unit. The speech behaviors of the child play a very significant role in furthering this aspect of developmental synchrony.

language aspects

The essential role of language in social and emotional development should be obvious. Language is the primary medium for social interactions between and among human beings. Starting at about age two, young children enter a period in which conversation, mostly with their mothers, provides information about themselves, about other people, and about the expectations and prohibitions of behavior. To return to our original definition—it is through language that children will further develop their perception of, and interaction with, self and others.

Child development occurs as a result of interactions between innate characteristics and environmental influences. Children develop in several areas simultaneously, preserving synchrony between these areas and between intrinsic needs and environmental conditions.

Hearing plays a key role in the development of speech skills as the child progresses through reflexive vocalization, purposeful vocalization, and communicative vocalization. The establishment of an association between the sounds and movements of speech is essential to this process.

As they develop cognitively, children assimilate sensory information and accomodate it into a personal, internal world model. Through the use of symbols that represent various aspects of this model, and rules for the arrangement of these symbols, children learn to communicate ideas to other people and to understand communications from others.

Nothing is more significant to the future of the child as a human being than social and emotional development. Hearing plays an important, but not essential, role in the initial stages of this development, and speech plays a more important, though still not essential, role in later stages. After the age of two years, proper social and emotional development are almost entirely dependent on the acquisition of adequate language skills.

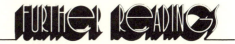

Grace Craig's *Human Development* (Prentice-Hall, Inc., Englewood Cliffs, N.J., 1976) is an example of the many excellent books available on this subject. It is a very readable text which presents summaries of various theories. As an introduction to the work of Jean Piaget, I suggest Piaget and Barbel Inhelder's *The Psychology of the Child* (Basic Books, New York, 1969).

The development of speech and language in normally hearing children receives excellent coverage in Peter and Jill De Villiers' *Language Acquisition* (1978) and *Early Language* (1979), (Harvard University Press, Cambridge, Mass.). The same material from the point of view of an audiologist and a teacher of the deaf is presented by

Richard and Laura Kretschmer in *Language Development and Intervention with the Hearing Impaired Child* (Univeristy Park Press, Baltimore, Md. 1978).

Burton White's book *The First Three Years* (Prentice-Hall, Inc., Englewood Cliffs, N.J., 1975) covers a particular age span, with special emphasis on the foundations of social and intellectual function. The development of speech is reviewed in many texts. As a starting point, I suggest Paula Menyuk's *Acquisition and Development of Language* (Prentice-Hall, Inc., Englewood Cliffs, N.J., 1971). Her more recent text on *Language and Maturation* (M.I.T. Press, Cambridge, Mass., 1977) is also recommended.

Edmund Critchley's *Speech Origins and Development* (Chas. C Thomas, Springfield, Ill., 1967) presents an interesting overview of cognition, language, and speech from an evolutionary point of view.

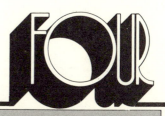

Impaired hearing

By its very nature, the hearing mechanism is sensitive and therefore vulnerable. From the results of various surveys we can estimate that out of every thousand babies, one or two will be born with serious hearing impairments and another twenty or thirty will have experienced hearing impairments by the time they are five years old.

The consequences of these impairments, the types of intervention that are possible, and the probable success of such intervention are determined by several factors. These include the location of the damage to the hearing mechanism, the cause of the damage, the time at which the damage occurs, the decibel loss of sensitivity, the stability of the threshold, and the coexistence of other impairments.

○ LOCATION OF DAMAGE (also known as *site of lesion*)

Hearing impairment can result from disorders in any of the three components of hearing, either singly or in combination.

conductive impairment

Conductive impairment occurs when the outer and middle ears do not transfer enough acoustic energy to the inner ear fluids. This may be due to blockage of the ear canal by congenital malformation, wax or foreign objects, or to abnormalities of the middle ear structures resulting from birth defects, injury, or disease. The commonest cause of conductive impairment in children is *otitis media*—or inflammation of the middle ear. At one stage this causes the middle ear space to fill with fluid, which limits vibrations of the tympanic membrane.

Conductive impairments reduce sensitivity by up to 50 dB or 60 dB, but they do not directly influence dynamic range, frequency range, discrimination capacity, attention, localization, recognition, or comprehension. If a conductive impairment persists or recurs, however, especially during early childhood, it can seriously affect perceptual development, causing behavioral and learning difficulties in the school years. In other words, conductive impairments can cause secondary neural impairments. Unlike sensory and neural problems, most conductive impairments can be treated successfully by medicine or surgery. If, for any reason, the loss of sensitivity is not reversible, the problem of energy transfer can largely be overcome by hearing aids.

It is very important for the teachers and parents of children with sensory and neural impairments to be alert to the signs of middle ear infections and to seek immediate treatment before an otherwise successful program of habilitative intervention is undermined.

sensory impairment

Sensory impairment occurs when the cochlea relays insufficient information about the sound patterns received from the middle ear. In adults, this is sometimes due to a chemical imbalance in the inner ear fluids that distorts the membranes and causes spontaneous stimulation of the acoustic and vestibular nerve endings. Although similar imbalances may occur in children, the most probable cause of sensory impairment is absence of some or all of the fine structures in the cochlea. These include the hair cells, the whole organ of corti, the membranes forming the cochlear partition, or the nerve fibers linking the hair cells to the auditory nerve.

The extent and severity of the damage to cochlear structures directly determines the loss of auditory sensitivity, which can range anywhere from a few decibels to over a hundred decibels. In extreme cases, the sense of hearing is lost completely, leaving the sense of touch as the only means of detecting sound. Since the cochlea separates sounds on the basis of frequency, it is quite possible for the loss of sensitivity to be different at different frequencies. In some cases, low frequency sensitivity is normal while high frequencies are completely inaudible, and the frequency range of hearing is therefore reduced.

Despite the loss of audibility for weak sounds, the perception of the loudness of strong sounds is usually normal. The result of this is a restricted dynamic range of intensity from threshold to discomfort—a condition known as *recruitment.*

Sensory impairments always involve a *loss of discrimination capacity* for frequency. The magnitude of this effect correlates highly with the loss of sensitivity. That is to say, the greater the decibel value of the hearing loss, the poorer the frequency discrimination. There can, however, be marked individual variations depending on the exact type of damage within the cochlea.

Another consequence of sensory impairment is that the cochlea's ability to prevent *interference among the frequencies of complex sounds* is reduced. The combination of this, the poor frequency discrimination, and the low dynamic intensity range severely limits the detail with which the cochlea can supply the brain with information about sound patterns.

When the fine structures within the cochlea are damaged, they do not heal themselves or regenerate, and they cannot be encouraged to do so with medicine, nor can they be repaired by surgery. The only "treatment" for sensory deafness is amplification. Using a hearing aid, we can compensate for the loss of sensitivity, providing it is not too great, and we can compress or limit the amplified signal to avoid causing discomfort. To a certain extent we can also balance the frequencies in the amplified signal to minimize the effects of masking within complex sounds, but it is important to realize that a hearing aid can do very little about the problem of discrimination capacity.

It is also important to realize that habilitative intervention cannot improve the sensitivity or the discrimination capacity of the cochlea. We can help children learn how to use the patterns of nerve impulses provided by their defective cochleas, but we cannot train the cochleas to produce more detailed patterns. The only aspect of cochlear function which appears to respond to training is dynamic intensity range. With extended listening experience, the cochlea is able to tolerate higher sound levels without registering discomfort. You should note that this effect does not transfer to an unaided cochlea. The child who learns to accept higher levels of amplification with only one ear will still have tolerance problems with the other.

neural impairment

Neural impairment is present when a child has difficulty processing the patterns of nerve impulses provided by the cochleas. This may result from direct damage to the neural mechanism or from the secondary effects of sensory and experiential deprivation.

If the neural mechanism is damaged at a low level (that is, close to the cochlea), there may be a loss of sensitivity and discrimination. In most cases of neural impairment, however, these functions are not affected. Instead, the child has difficulties with auditory attention, awareness, memory, recognition, association, and comprehension.

When the auditory processing problems are severe, they can cause children to behave as if they have a loss of sensitivity. This phenomenon creates difficulties of diagnosis. It is also responsible for the improvements of threshold that are sometimes observed as a result of training or quasi-medical treatment.

In fact, neither medicine, surgery, nor hearing aids have much to offer in the treatment of neural impairments. Where remediation is possible, it will be accomplished by habilitative intervention. Where it is not possible, the problems must be circumvented—also by habilitative intervention. Determining which problems are reversible and which are not is the role of diagnostic teaching. There is considerable evidence to suggest that the longer we delay intervention, the more likely we are to encounter irreversible problems.

sensorineural impairment

In practice, the division between sensory and neural impairments is often difficult to determine. There are several reasons for this. One is that the first stages of the neural mechanism are inside the cochlea. A second is that many of the causes of deafness produce damage to both the sensory and the neural mechanisms. A third is that neural impairments are usually present as a secondary consequence of sensory impairment. A fourth is that many of the behavioral consequences of sensory and neural deafness are similar. For these reasons, it is usual to refer to all nonconductive impairments as *sensorineural.* The reason I have made the distinction in the present book is to emphasize that prosthetic and habilitative intervention have different targets. We use hearing aids to deal with sensory problems and habilitation to deal with neural problems.

section summary

Conductive impairments reduce the efficiency with which sound energy is transferred from the surrounding air to the inner ear fluids. Most of them can be treated successfully by medicine or surgery. Sensory impairments reduce the sensitivity, dynamic range, and discrimination capacity of the cochlea. Changes of sensitivity and dynamic range can be compensated by hearing aids if the impairment is not too severe, but there is no way to restore the lost discrimination capacity. Neural impairments cause difficulties of attention, awareness, memory, recognition, association, and comprehension. They may be caused by direct damage to the neural mechanism or indirect damage resulting from understimulation. Habilitative intervention can reverse some of these problems and develop ways of circumventing those which are irreversible.

○ CAUSES OF HEARING IMPAIRMENT

The known causes of hearing impairment in young children fall into four major categories: heredity, disease, drugs, and trauma.

heredity

Roughly half of the serious hearing impairments in young children are the result of defective genes inherited from one or both parents. Genes may be thought of as chemical instructions for the assembly of an organism. Several thousand genes are required for the assembly of a human being. These are arranged in pairs in the chromosomes of each cell of our bodies.

At the moment of conception, a child receives one member of each pair from the mother and the other member from the father. This may seem confusing, since two sets of instructions are available, but in practice one member of each pair dominates the other. Sometimes this is the one inherited from the mother, and sometimes it is the one inherited from the father.

Each person carries a handful of defective genes but if two people are selected at random, the chances that they will have the same defective genes are very small. Thus there is a good chance that children will inherit at least one "good" gene in each of the pairs they receive from their parents. In most cases a normal gene will dominate a defective gene, and no harm will be done.

Problems arise under two circumstances. The first occurs when the defective gene dominates the normal gene. The second occurs when the child receives two defective genes in a pair. If these genes are involved in the assembly or nourishment of the hearing mechanism, the child will inherit a hearing impairment. In the first case it has been acquired by *dominant inheritance,* in the second case by *recessive inheritance.* From the results of various genetic studies it is known that there are several different dominant genes and several different recessive genes that can cause hearing impairment.

When a child is hearing-impaired by simple dominant inheritance, it is certain that one parent is hearing-impaired, and there is a 50 percent chance that each of his or her siblings will be hearing-impaired. When a child is hearing-impaired by simple recessive inheritance, neither parent need be hearing-impaired, but there is a good chance that some of his or her siblings will be hearing-impaired. The occurence of recessively inherited hearing impairments is greater in children whose parents were directly related (for example, second or third cousins) before marriage.

The foregoing is a simplified description of inheritance. The problem is greatly complicated by such factors as partial dominance, genetic damage caused by chemicals or radiation, and sex-linked inheritance.

Inherited hearing impairments can take several forms. Sometimes the cochlea fails to develop or develops abnormally. Sometimes the cochlea develops normally, but the fine structures are missing or defective. Sometimes the cochlea and its fine structures develop normally but then degenerate because of imperfections in the systems that should nourish and support them. And finally, the cochlea and its support systems may be adequate for normal everyday demands but are unable to tolerate extra demands caused by illnesses, drugs, and excessive noise.

There are also inherited hearing impairments in which the external and middle ear structures fail to develop or develop abnormally, and you should note that in some cases, the defective gene may simultaneously reveal itself in features that seem to have nothing to do with hearing (for example, skeletal characteristics and pigmentation of the eyes, skin, and hair).

From a habilitative point of view, the important characteristics of inherited hearing impairment are as follows:

1. Direct neural impairment is not usually involved. This means that if habilitative procedures are begun early, the prognosis is good.

2. Although the time of acquisition of the genetic defect is at the moment of conception, the time of acquisition of the hearing impairment can vary. It is quite common for the child with inherited hearing impairment to be born with perfect hearing and to lose it during the first few days, months, or years of life.

3. If the genetic defect is slight, the hearing impairment may not appear until triggered by some other causative factor such as illness, drugs, or trauma. In such cases it is impossible to specify a single cause.

4. A high percentage of hearing impairments whose cause is listed as unknown are probably the result of recessive inheritance.

disease

Congenital hearing impairments can be the result of viral infections contracted by the mother during pregnancy. The best known example is rubella, or German measles, but other infections are believed to have similar effects. The exact nature and severity of the damage caused to the developing embryo depends on its stage of development—the most critical period being the first three months of gestation. If hearing is affected, there are usually both sensory and neural impairments. Sometimes conductive impairments occur as well.

Incompatibility between the Rh factor in the blood of the mother and that of the child may cause the mother's system to develop antibodies that destroy the child's red blood cells, leading to severe anemia and jaundice. The resulting loss of nutrients to the cochlea, as well as the high levels of toxic pigments in the bloodstream, can produce both sensory and neural hearing impairments.

You should note that both rubella and Rh incompatibility were brought under control in the late 1960s as a result of developments in immunology. Nevertheless, they may still make sporadic appearances as causes of hearing impairment, and there are other diseases that have similar effects.

Of the diseases that can be contracted by children themselves, with hearing impairment as a possible consequence, the best known example is meningitis. This is an inflammation of the meninges—a membrane surrounding the brain. It can be caused by both viral and bacterial agents. If these invade the inner ear, they lead to partial or complete destruction of the hair cells in both the cochlea and the vestibular mechanism. There can also be damage to the neural mechanism of hearing. In extreme instances the deafness is total and even when there is a small amount of residual hearing, the discrimination capacity of the cochlea is often much poorer than when the damage is caused by other agents. Another characteristic of hearing impairments caused by meningitis is that the auditory sensitivity can go through a period of marked fluctuation for several months after the illness.

Other childhood diseases, such as measles and mumps, can cause sensory deafness, especially if an unusually high fever is involved. In such cases, there is probably an interaction between the illness and individual suscepti-bility to hearing impairment based on genetic differences.

The commonest cause of hearing impairment in children is otitis media. This is an inflammation of the middle ear caused by failure of the eustachian tube and/or an infection of the middle ear cavity. The result is a conductive impairment that is usually reversible.

drugs

As in the case of diseases, certain drugs may affect hearing if in-gested by a mother during pregnancy, others if ingested by the child after birth. Organisms and drugs that injure a developing embryo are known as *teratogens* (literally—*monster makers*). These were brought to the public's at-tention by the Thalidomide tragedy of the early 1960s, but Thalidomide is only one of several drugs whose teratogenic effects are known or suspected. These include certain aborting agents. The nature and severity of the effects of these drugs depends upon the stage of embryonic development at the time they are ingested. Hearing impairments caused by them can be conduc-tive, sensory, or neural.

Among drugs with a direct *ototoxic* (literally—*ear poisoning*) effect, the best known is dihydrostreptomycin. This is a powerful antibiotic that may be used to treat a life-threatening illness at the risk of damaging hearing. Its effect is to destroy hair cells, and the resulting impairment is therefore sensory.

trauma

Under the heading of trauma I am including all agents other than drugs or disease that either interfere with the development of the hearing mechanism or damage it after it has developed.

Malnutrition and radiation can seriously affect a developing embryo, impaired hearing being one of several possible consequences. A prolonged and difficult labor or premature delivery may deprive the child of oxygen and nutrients long enough for the sensory and neural mechanisms of hear-ing to suffer permanent damage. This can also occur as a result of seizures in the young child. Other damaging agents are severe head blows and extremely loud noises (for example, explosions). These can cause both conductive and sensory impairments. Damage of the tympanic membrane and middle ear structures by a foreign object such as a hairpin or twig is unlikely but does occur from time to time.

relevance to habilitation

Knowledge of causation can prepare a teacher for the types of problems that are likely to be met in habilitative intervention. It is particularly important, for example, to be aware of the possibility of primary neural impairment and to be ready with alternative approaches if the child's progress does not follow the "text book" (this or any other).

You should also realize that when a previously intact neural mechanism is damaged through oxygen deprivation, for example, any neural organization occurring up to that time may be nullified. In a sense, the child's brain must return to a prenatal developmental stage, and he or she will require several months to reorganize. This will cause a delay of all developmental milestones, including those related to habilitation.

During a thirty-year period beginning in the mid-1940s, there were significant changes in medicine that had a marked effect on the patterns of causation among hearing-impaired children. Many known diseases were brought under control, virtually eliminating them as a cause of deafness. At the same time, however, improvements in obstetric practice resulted in the survival of many infants who previously would have died. These children frequently have sensorineural hearing impairments as well as other impairments that affect their ability to learn. Habilitative intervention with these children can be very difficult.

section summary

Hearing impairments are caused by heredity, disease, drugs, and trauma. Within each category there are causes that interfere with embryonic development as well as causes that damage an otherwise intact hearing mechanism. Knowledge of causation can be useful to teachers and should be taken into account when planning intervention.

For purposes of reference, Figure 4–1 shows a list of causes, together with information on place of damage. Also included is information on time of acquisition and severity of hearing loss—topics that are discussed in the next two sections.

○ TIME OF ACQUISITION

The impact of a hearing impairment depends partly on the age at which it is acquired. This is not surprising since hearing is itself a learned

CAUSE		TYPE			TIME ACQUIRED			HEARING LOSS					STABILITY			ADDITIONAL IMPAIRMENTS
General Cause:	Specific Example:	Conductive	Sensory	Neural	Before birth	Around birth	After birth	Mild	Moderate	Severe	Profound	Total	Stable	Progressive	Fluctuating	
GENETIC	Dominant	○	●		●	●	●	●	●	●	●	●	●	○		
	Recessive	○	●		●	●	●	●	●	●	●	●	●	○		
DISEASE	Rubella	○	●	●	●			●	●	●	●		●			●
	Rh factor		●	●	●			●	●	●	●		●			●
	Meningitis		●	○			●			●	●	●	●	○	○	○
	Mumps		●				●			●	●	●	●			
	Otitis media	●					●	●	●	●					●	
DRUGS	Teratogens	●	●	●	●			●	●	●	●		●			●
	Ototoxins		●				●			●	●	●	●			
TRAUMA	In utero	●	●	●	●			●	●	●	●		●			●
	Prematurity		●	●		●		●	●	●	●		●			●
	At birth		●	●		●		●	●	●	●		●			●
	Anoxia		●	●		●	○	●	●	●	●		●			●
	Noise		●				●	●	●	●			●			
	Head blow	●	●				●	●	●	●	●	●	●			○
	Impacted wax	●					●	●	●						●	

● = Probable   ○ = Possible

FIGURE 4–1 Causes and characteristics of hearing impairments in young children.

skill which plays a critical role in development. There are, however, some common misunderstandings about this issue that require clarification.

congenital does not mean inherited

The term *congenital* refers to any condition that was present at the moment of birth. Congenital hearing impairments may result from heredity, blood incompatibility, teratogens, or traumatic delivery.

The first of these four—heredity—does not *always* produce congenital hearing impairment. In this connection you must distinguish between time of acquisition of the genetic defect and time of acquisition of the resulting impairment. The genetic defect is acquired at the moment of conception. The hearing impairment can be acquired at any time of life. As I pointed out in an earlier section, it is not uncommon for babies to be born with perfectly normal hearing and to lose it during the first few days, months, or years of life as a result of heredity.

all prelingual impairments are not equal

It is common to distinguish between hearing impairments that occur before language develops and those that occur after language develops. While it is true that there are important qualitative differences between the child who loses his or her hearing at age eighteen months and the one who loses it at age five years, the situation is by no means as simple as this binary classification suggests.

It is a mistake to assume that language development begins when the child starts using one or two word utterances. Language development begins at birth. The baby who hears normally for the first twelve months of life and then loses hearing has already travelled part way along the path of language development and is in a better position to benefit from habilitative intervention than if he or she had been born with the same hearing impairment.

In fact, children retain whatever skills they have consolidated at the time of a sensory impairment. They may lose skills that they have developed but not yet consolidated, though immediate habilitative intervention can help to preserve them.

○ DEGREE OF HEARING LOSS

The auditory sensitivity of a hearing-impaired child plays a large part in determining developmental progress, either with or without intervention. This is particularly true in cases of purely sensory loss. We cannot, of course, predict the exact progress of an individual child solely from a knowledge of pure tone thresholds, but we can estimate the likelihood of his or her achieving various levels of performance.

hearing loss groups

The relationship between hearing loss and developmental progress is determined primarily by the way an impairment affects the audibility of conversational speech. This you will recall covers an intensity range of 30 dB to 60 dB above the normal threshold of hearing. Two other factors are also important. The first is that in cases of sensory deafness, there is a steady decrease of discrimination capacity with increasing hearing loss. The second is that wearable hearing aids can seldom provide more than 60 dB of amplification, this limit being set by problems of acoustic feedback.

As a result of these three factors, audibility of conversational speech, discrimination capacity, and amplification limit, children with sensory impairments fall into five, qualitatively different, groups:

Group I—Hearing losses 15 dB to 30 dB These children retain full audibility of conversational speech and develop spoken language skills spontaneously. If the threshold is stable, the effects of the impairment are slight, and the hearing loss can be described as *mild.*

Group II—Hearing losses 31 dB to 60 dB These children retain partial audibility of conversational speech and develop spoken language skills spontaneously but imperfectly. Hearing aids can restore full audibility of speech and permit use of the children's good discrimination capacity. With appropriate intervention, most of the speech and language problems of these children can be eliminated. Their hearing loss may be described as *moderate.*

Group III—Hearing losses 61 dB to 90 dB These children do not hear normal conversational speech and do not develop spoken language skills spontaneously. Without amplification and habilitation, they function as if totally deaf. Modern hearing aids can give them full audibility of conversational speech, however, and permit use of their good discrimination capacities. Such problems as these children have with discrimination are limited mainly to voice quality and place of articulation of consonants. Thus, with appropriate intervention, they can use hearing as their primary modality for the acquisition of spoken language skills. Their hearing losses may be described as *severe.*

Group IV—Hearing losses 91 dB to 120 dB These children do not hear normal conversational speech, and even with modern hearing aids, we can restore only partial audibility. This limitation, combined with poor discrimination capacity, makes it difficult for hearing to become the primary modality for acquiring spoken language skills. The main value of hearing to these children is in learning to recognize and produce the prosodic features of speech, and as a supplement to lipreading, in learning to recognize and produce the segmental features. Their hearing losses may be described as *profound.*

Group V—Hearing losses 121 dB or more These children do not hear conversational speech, with or without hearing aids. All indications are that they perceive sound, not with the sense of hearing, but with the sense of touch. If they are to acquire spoken language skills, they must use the sense of vision as their primary modality for learning. Their losses may be described as *total.*

borderlines

Within each of the groups just defined, there are significant differences. A child with a 100 dB hearing loss, for example, stands to gain more from prosthetic-habilitative intervention than does one with a 115 dB hearing loss. You should also note that the group boundaries, which I have placed at 30, 60, 90 and 120 dB, are by no means as clear-cut as the foregoing presentation suggests. For this reason I refer to hearing losses within ± 5 dB of these boundaries as *borderline.* For example, a loss of 93 dB is *borderline severe to profound* and a loss of 115 dB is *borderline profound to total.*

deaf and hard-of-hearing

The terms *deaf* and *hard-of-hearing* originated in simpler days when less was known about hearing impairment and when hearing aids and habilitation were not available. We still use these terms although the limitations of a binary classification have become something of an embarrassment. My own preference is to use deaf and hard-of-hearing when referring to an individual's speech perception ability (See Chapter One.) Thus, without amplification, children with moderate hearing losses will be functionally hard-of-hearing, while children with severe, profound, and total losses will be deaf. With amplification and appropriate intervention, children with severe losses (and some with profound losses) can become functionally hard-of-hearing, in the sense that they can understand what is said to them by hearing, using vision as a support.

neural impairments and multiple handicaps

I must stress again that the classification of hearing losses, based on sensitivity, is most meaningful when applied to children with purely sensory losses. The value of pure tone threshold as a predictor of performance becomes weaker as we encounter primary neural impairments or additional problems of perceptual and symbolic function.

section summary

Children with sensory impairments fall into five qualitatively different groups, depending on their ability to detect the sounds of normal conversational speech. Those with mild losses (15 dB to 30 dB) retain full audibility, those with moderate losses (31 dB to 60 dB) retain partial audibility, and those with losses of over 60 dB retain no audibility. Without hearing aids these groups could be labelled *slightly hard-of-hearing, hard-of-hearing,* and *deaf* respectively. Modern hearing aids can restore full audibility of conversational speech to children with moderate losses (31 dB to 60 dB) and severe losses (61 dB to 90 dB) and partial audibility to those with profound losses (91 dB to 120 dB). If the loss is total (121 dB or more), conversational speech remains inaudible, even with hearing aids. The effect of early amplification and appropriate intervention is to make children with severe losses (and even some with profound losses) functionally hard-of-hearing. The majority of those with profound losses, and all those with total losses, remain deaf, however, in the sense that their primary input modality for acquisition of spoken language skills is vision, though many of them can make significant use of hearing in a supportive role. These observations lose their validity when primary neural impairments or additional handicaps are present. (See also Table 4–1.)

○ STABILITY

Hearing losses fall into three categories on the basis of threshold stability. In *stable* losses, the threshold remains constant over time; in *progressive* losses, the threshold deteriorates steadily (or stepwise) over time; in *fluctuating* losses, the threshold varies up and down over time.

TABLE 4.1
Hearing Loss: Classification and Characteristics

Group	Threshold Range*	Description of Hearing Loss	WITHOUT AMPLIFICATION			WITH AMPLIFICATION		
			Audibility of Conversational Speech	Discrimination Capacity for Speech	Learning Modality	Audibility of Conversational Speech	Discrimination Capacity	Learning Modality
I	15–30 dB	Mild	Normal	Normal	Auditory	Normal	Normal	Auditory
II	31–60 dB	Moderate	Partial	Almost normal	Auditory w. support from vision	Normal	Almost normal	Auditory
III	61–90 dB	Severe	None	Irrelevant	Visual	Normal	Good**	Auditory w. support from vision
IV	91–120 dB	Profound	None	Irrelevant	Visual	Partial	Poor***	Visual w. support from audition
V	121 dB or more	Total	None	Irrelevant	Visual	None	Irrelevant	Visual

* Average of pure tone thresholds at 500, 1000 and 2000 Hz in dBHL using the standard for normal threshold set by the American National Standards Institute (ANSI) in 1969.

** Main problems are with discrimination of voice quality differences and place of articulation of consonants.

*** Main benefits of hearing are in recognition and control of rhythm and intonation and discrimination of certain vowel differences.

stable losses

Obviously, the most desirable condition (after normal hearing) is a stable loss. The performance of the hearing mechanism is reliable and predictable, and it is safe for the child to incorporate sound into his or her perceptual development and to give it priority when appropriate.

progressive losses

It is disturbing for children to lose, or suffer a deterioration in, a sensory modality on which they have come to rely. If the progression is slow, however, there is time to adapt to the changes, and the benefits of having started with better hearing will always be apparent. Progressive losses are commonest in cases of sensory impairment caused by hereditary factors.

fluctuating losses

Postmeningitic children often go through a period of fluctuating loss for five or six months following the illness. Even after this time there may still be progression.

By far the most common cause of fluctuating loss, however, is otitis media. The consequences of a fluctuating loss caused by recurrent ear infections are serious but easily overlooked. The basic problem is that because their hearing is unreliable and unpredictable, children do not integrate sound adequately into their general perceptual development and they do not give sound the priority it deserves. They, therefore, develop difficulties of auditory attention which may further lead to problems of auditory memory and recognition, even after the thresholds have returned to normal.

hearing aids and stability of hearing loss

Children with moderate, severe, and profound hearing losses use hearing aids to obtain much of their acoustic information. If the hearing aids are not worn regularly, or if they are not maintained in full working order, these children suffer artificially induced fluctuating losses. Only if the hearing aid becomes a reliable, predictable, and integral component of the child's hearing mechanism can we expect sound to play its optimal role in development. Some authorities go so far as to argue that changing from personal hearing aids to classroom hearing aids and back again is equivalent to inflicting a fluctuating hearing loss on the child and works against auditory development.

The population of hearing-impaired infants and preschoolers presents a wide variety of characteristics and needs. Hearing impairments differ in terms of location, cause, time of acquisition, degree of loss, and stability of threshold, and they may occur alone or in combination with other impairments. Each of these factors influences the consequences of the hearing impairment, the choice of intervention strategy, and the probable outcome of intervention. Each factor may act alone or it may interact with other factors, both auditory and nonauditory. For ease of reference, much of the information presented in this chapter is summarized in Figure 4–1 and Table 4–1.

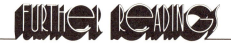

As very readable introductions to hearing impairments and their evaluation, I suggest Frederick N. Martin's *Introduction to Audiology*—second edition, (Prentice-Hall, Inc., Englewood Cliffs, N.J., 1981) and Jerry Northern and Marion Downs' *Hearing in Children*—second edition, (Williams & Wilkins, Baltimore, Md., 1978). Although a multiauthored book, Martin's *Pediatric Audiology* (Prentice-Hall, Inc., Englewood Cliffs, NJ., 1978) is very cohesive. Another multiauthored book, less cohesive but still a valuable source of information, is Burton Jaffe's *Hearing Loss in Children* (University Park Press, Baltimore, Md., 1977). If you wish to delve a little more deeply into genetics, I recommend Lucille Whaley's *Understanding Inherited Disorders* (C. V. Mosby, St. Louis, Mo., 1974).

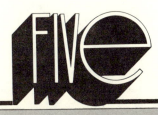

Development of the hearing-impaired child

In Chapter Four we saw how hearing impairments differ in terms of degree, cause, type, time of acquisition, stability, and the presence of other problems. All of these factors help to determine how an impairment affects development, as do such things as the personality of the child, the education and cultural background of the parents, their economic situation, and their familiarity with hearing impairment. So complicated is this topic that it would be impossible to cover it in a single chapter. I have therefore chosen to describe the development of a particular kind of child. This is the child with a severe, profound, or total sensory hearing loss and normally hearing parents who have never previously met a hearing-impaired person. This description is followed by an indication of the changes that are introduced as some of the critical factors are varied. The chapter ends with a discussion of the essential components of habilitative intervention and of various philosophies of approach.

○ EFFECTS OF THE HEARING IMPAIRMENT ON THE CHILD

Each of the developmental areas discussed in Chapter Four is affected by the exclusion of sound from the developing child's experience of the world.

perceptual development

The perceptual development of profoundly deaf children proceeds on schedule despite the missing sensory dimension. They are aroused and alerted by sensory stimuli; they pay attention to sensory stimuli; they develop a knowledge of space and time; and they establish a world model of permanent objects and predictable events. The difference, of course, is that acoustic events play no part in this process. These children are alerted by tactile, olfactory, or visual sensations but not by auditory sensations; they learn about space and time through motoric, tactile, and visual exploration but get no assistance from sound; and they recognize objects and events on the basis of tactile, olfactory, and visual patterns but not from auditory patterns.

The effects of the hearing impairment on behavior become increasingly obvious as the children get older. At first they may sleep better because they are not disturbed by noises, but this "benefit" is offset by the fact that when upset, they are not soothed by the sound of mother's voice. At a few months of age it will be clear that they are not receiving acoustic clues to their parents' entry into the room, although they may compensate by feeling the vibrations of footsteps or noticing shadows on the wall. Between six and nine months, their failure to turn when called or to look for the source of a sound will be obvious to objective observers.

At some stage in the developmental process, the hearing-impaired child will be fitted with hearing aids. These will make many environmental sounds audible but will by no means establish the perceptual skills that would have been present had the child been born with normal hearing. There are several reasons for this. One is the poor discrimination capacity of the defective cochlea. Another is the aid's inherent lack of reliability. Batteries die, faults develop, earmolds become plugged, and aids are taken off at bedtime. Between them, the hearing aid and the cochlea may not provide the neural mechanism with the consistent and detailed auditory information on which the development of perceptual skills relies.

The biggest deterrents to auditory development, however, are the aftereffects of sensory deprivation and the lack of developmental synchrony. There is a lot of evidence to support the contention that neural mechanisms develop imperfectly, or even deteriorate, when they are not stimulated. In addition, for profoundly deaf children who first receive a hearing aid at age two or three years, sound is not a source of information—it is an intrusion. Their perceptual world does not have an auditory component; their attention mechanism has no priority for auditory sensations, and differences of signal at the right and left ears do not have any spatial significance. It is not enough to say that these children must learn to hear. They must do something much more difficult. They must unlearn some of the perceptual skills they have already developed and relearn them with hearing as an integral component. Moreover, they must do so with auditory systems that are damaged, and with the help of prosthetic devices of questionable reliability. This is not impossible, but neither is it easy or automatic.

speech development

During the first few months of life, profoundly deaf children vocalize reflexively. They may even do some purposeful babbling as they explore the resulting tactile and kinesthetic sensations. However, in the absence of auditory feedback and without auditory models from their parents, this activity will soon be abandoned in favor of more rewarding ones. From about nine months of age, the vocal output of profoundly deaf children is limited to the reflexive acts of crying and laughing.

Once hearing aids are fitted, the same factors hinder speech development as hinder auditory development. These are the limited discrimination capacity of the defective cochlea, the poor reliability of the hearing aid, neurological (and also neuromuscular) consequences of understimulation, and the frustrations of developmental asynchrony. If profoundly deaf children are to develop speech skills in a natural (that is, auditory) manner, they must pass through the stages of reflexive, purposive, and imitative vocalization before they can begin to use speech for communication. They must develop the underlying auditory skills, and they must establish the auditory-motor associations that are the basis of controlled speech. Unless the aids are fitted at a very early age, these children must engage in activities that are inappropriate to their general level of motoric, cognitive, and social development and that may therefore be unrewarding and frustrating.

cognitive and linguistic development

Lack of hearing does not interfere significantly with cognitive development during the first two years of life. Profoundly deaf toddlers establish world models with perceptual and conceptual categories. There is, however, no access to these models through acoustic inputs, and this becomes a serious problem when a need emerges for the labelling of conceptual categories. The verbal symbols used by the parents simply do not exist for their children. It is true that facial movements can be seen during speech, but these movements are so inconsistent, so similar, and so irrelevant that the children do not pay attention to them. Even if they did attend to and attempt to imitate their parents' speech activities, the children's efforts would not produce audible sounds. Why should they? Visible speech movements are almost trivial by-products of the essential speech process. Most of the important speech activities (for example, breathing, laryngeal function, change in status of the velum, and movements of the tongue) are as invisible to profoundly deaf children as the acoustic results are inaudible.

How then do these children respond to the inner drive to externalize and communicate the results of their general cognitive development and immediate thinking processes? They do it through gesture and mime, and their parents respond in the same way. Once a gesture has been used several times, it functions as a symbol that can be traded back and forth, its referent being understood by the parties concerned. For a while this works well as it permits parents and child to communicate about the immediate and the familiar. There are, however, some crippling limitations. This gestural communication does not provide the children with access to the language used between their parents and among the other people with whom they come into contact; each symbolic gesture must be made up from scratch, and most serious of all, there are no rules for combining symbols—there is no grammar by which "old" symbols can be rearranged to express "new" ideas.

Without further intervention, profoundly deaf children remain at a primitive and concrete level of communication and their cognitive development is unable to benefit from the expanded horizons to which language is the normal access.

One component of intervention is the fitting of hearing aids, but this will not provide an immediate or simple solution. Basic auditory and speech skills must be established before verbal language acquisition can occur, and even then the children will need to be engaged in communicative interchanges that are more appropriate to an earlier stage of development and that may again be intrinsically unrewarding for both children and parents.

social and emotional development

During the first two years of life, a lack of hearing can have significant effects on children's perception of themselves and others. For example, there are no auditory clues to their parents' approach and unless warned by footsteps or shadows, they may repeatedly be surprised by the parents' precipitous appearance. Similarly, when parents leave, the children do not have auditory clues that reassure the normal child of their continued existence. The mother-child bond must develop without the benefits of acoustic contact. Profoundly deaf children are not calmed by their mother's voices, and they do not discover the power of control that comes from a normal baby's first attempts at "conversation." Yet another problem is that as their world model expands to include emotional states—their own and other people's—deaf children do not have the benefit of the cues that are normally provided by tone of voice and intonation pattern. However, none of these problems is insurmountable. Hearing is a valuable factor in the early stages of social and emotional development, but it is not indispensable.

When profoundly deaf children reach the age at which verbal language would normally become the primary medium for interaction with their parents, the failure to acquire skills in this area has profound social and emotional effects. They are frustrated by their limited ability to externalize thoughts and wishes and by their lack of control over the social environment. They perceive themselves as being acted upon more than acting and may compensate by developing rigid and manipulative behaviors. It is, of course, normal for a child to enter a period of negativism and rigidity between the second and third birthday, but with proper management and adequate language development, this stage is passed in a few months and a *social contract* is established between child and parents. The profoundly deaf child and his or her family must also establish a contract, but in the absence of language its terms are likely to be extremely unfavorable to one or other of the parties concerned. This phenomenon will repeat itself as the child's social environment expands to include other adults and children.

I must stress that the issue here is not specifically the lack of hearing, but the failure to develop language—a process to which hearing would normally be the key. Children who do not have a viable language system by the time they are three or four years old, or do not acquire one soon thereafter, are in serious social and emotional jeopardy.

○ EFFECTS OF THE HEARING IMPAIRMENT ON THE PARENTS

We must remember that the developmental process is one in which child and parents share the roles of actors and reactors. The children's hearing loss, or more exactly their failure to develop auditory, speech, and language skills, affects their parents—sometimes dramatically—causing them to change their own behaviors. This, in turn, alters the children's social and communicative environment and further influences their development.

discovery of the hearing loss

It is the mother (or her surrogate) who spends most time with the young baby and who, therefore, has the greatest opportunity for observation and interaction. Not surprisingly, therefore, it is usually the mother who first suspects a hearing problem. The first clues may be the baby's failure to startle to loud sounds, or to show awareness of people's presence from sound alone. If the mother shares her concerns with her husband, her own parents, or her pediatrician, she may be told that she is worrying unnecessarily. This opinion is very acceptable, and there is supporting evidence. Sometimes profoundly deaf babies do startle; sometimes they do turn or quiet when mother enters the room; sometimes they do turn to look for the source of a sound. They are, of course, responding to tactile and visual clues, but the parents do not realize that this is so.

Although, for the time being, the mother tries to suppress her concerns, the seeds of doubt have been sown, and this may change her feelings about, and her behavior towards her baby. Her fears are a discord in an otherwise harmonious relationship.

The baby's failure to babble beyond six or seven months of age affects the mother's own verbal behavior. At first, like all mothers, she talks to her baby as though every word is understood. This is instinctive, but its continuation requires the reward of the baby's own verbal efforts. In the absence of this feedback, the mother talks to her baby less and less.

At about eight or nine months of age, the deaf child is sitting unsupported and showing great interest in the physical and social environment. The disparity between visual responsiveness and auditory responsiveness now becomes apparent to both mother and father, who are likely to spend a lot of time "testing" with the loudest noisemakers they can find—typically spoons and saucepans. Concerns are again expressed to the pediatrician. Whether he or she refers the child for professional evaluation or attempts to dispel the parents' concerns, depends on training, experience, and orientation. Since the rubella epidemic of the 1960s, more and more pediatricians have become informed about hearing impairments in young children and about the possibilities for evaluation, amplification, and early intervention. There is also more awareness of this subject among the general public. In spite of this, it is still the exception, rather than the rule, for intervention to begin before the child is one year old, and it is common for a second birthday to pass without the problem having been professionally identified.

Sooner or later, however, the child will be seen by a competent evaluation team, and the parents will be told, "Your baby is deaf."

mourning

Even though the professional verdict is only a confirmation of what was already suspected, its impact is severe, and the parents must pass through a predictable sequence of reactions and adjustments. This process is what we call *mourning*. It has much in common with people's reactions to a physical disaster, the death of a loved one, or the diagnosis of an incurable disease—in fact, any serious loss. In an earlier chapter we discussed cognitive development in terms of a world model. Essentially, people in crisis are faced with events and experiences for which there are no places in their world models. It takes time for them to assimilate and accommodate to the new circumstances. Hopefully they grow and mature as a result.

I shall discuss the stages of the mourning process in turn:

1. *Shock* The state of shock is a natural defense mechanism. At a physical level it diminishes the effects of injury. At an emotional level it protects the individual from information which is unacceptable. The processes of recognition and comprehension that normally provide access to the world of reality are temporarily shut down. It is no use trying to explain anything to the parents of a deaf child when they are in this condition. This is no time for a comparison of conductive and sensorineural impairment, an explanation of how a hearing aid works, or exhortations to enrich the child's language environment. They quite literally will not hear you. They may detect your speech sounds, but they will not interpret them.

2. *Denial* As the protective effects of shock wear off, the parents enter a period during which they attempt to hold on to their world model and to change reality. They question the diagnosis. They do more home testing, seizing on the slightest evidence of auditory responsiveness as "proof" that their child can hear. They seek another opinion, and perhaps another, and another. If they accept that their child has a hearing impairment, they may refuse to accept the fact that it is incurable. Some parents never quite leave this stage. They continue to hope for a cure. They grasp at acupuncture, cochlear implants, new hearing aids—anything that promises to restore to them the "normal" child they lost and for whom there is still a place in their world model. You should be aware of the fact that for many parents, the habilitative process is also one from which they expect their child to emerge "whole."

3. *Anger* When the parents begin to accept reality and to change their perceptions, they do not do so willingly. They are understandably angry. Their life has taken a direction that is not of their own choosing. Like the child without language, they feel acted upon rather than acting. This anger can be self-directed, or it can be directed at the child, the spouse, the doctor, you the teacher, fate, or God. Closely allied with this anger is a desire to apportion blame.

4. *Passive Acceptance* As the futility of anger becomes apparent, there may be a period of passive acceptance, similar to depression. The parents are grieving the loss of a perfect child, and they feel helpless. It is as though they are entering a tunnel with no light at the end. They feel sorry for themselves and for their child.

5. *Constructive Acceptance* The final stage is one of constructive acceptance in which the parents come to know their child as he or she is. They slowly accept their own responsibility for learning about deafness and for adapting their behaviors so that they can meet the child's unfolding needs and be prepared to make difficult decisions that will affect his or her future.

A theme which pervades the mourning process is that of *guilt.* This is a complicated and disabling emotion. The parents may feel guilty at having caused the hearing impairment or at having caused the damaged child to exist. They may feel guilty because they are angry or because they feel inadequate to the task ahead of them. I believe that guilt can run even deeper than this—that it can arise from the conflict between the parents' instinctive rejection of a child who is "different" and their equally instinctive desire to accept and nurture the same child because he or she is their own.

The net effect of shock, denial, anger, depression, and guilt is one of impotence. Until the parents have worked their way through to positive acceptance, they are incapable of meeting their child's basic social and emotional needs—let alone the special needs that the hearing impairment has revealed. The duration of this adjustment period can vary from a few weeks to several years. For some parents it is a permanent condition. In most cases the mother, being closer to the problem, progresses more rapidly than the father. If the disparity is severe, it can drive a wedge between the parents and contribute to a breakup of the family. Equally dangerous is the situation in which the mother throws herself wholeheartedly into the management of the hearing-impaired child to the exclusion of other family roles and emotional relationships, perhaps because of some deep unmet need in herself.

You should also note that the mourning sequence can be replayed several times in the parents' lives. As the child gets older, and the implications of the hearing impairment are seen more clearly, the parents may return to states of denial and anger. Each time, however, it should be possible to progress through this sequence faster and more easily.

I should make one more point before leaving this topic. The process we have just described is in no way pathological. It is a normal, inevitable, and indeed healthy reaction to a serious loss. One of your roles is to provide support during the early stages of mourning so that the parents will understand and come to terms with their own reactions and conflicts and begin to deal effectively with their child's needs. Progress of the child is absolutely dependent on the mediation of his or her parents, but you will gain nothing by trying to bypass, ignore, or hurry through the mourning process. On the contrary, you will be creating yet another kind of developmental asynchrony and storing up even greater problems for the future.

○ EFFECTS OF PARENTS' REACTIONS ON THE CHILD

Changes in parent behavior obviously alter the environment of the child and therefore affect development.

perceptual

The homemade testing that parents do when they first suspect a hearing impairment, and during the denial stage of mourning, is liable to slow down auditory development. This is particularly true after a profoundly deaf child has been fitted with hearing aids. Since these loud noises the parents are making have no relevance to the child's immediate interests and activities, they will be ignored rather than attended to, and this behavior may spread over into potentially meaningful sounds.

Once they are convinced that their child is hearing-impaired, parents often withhold useful sources of auditory stimulation. For example, they may deliberately choose not to provide noise-making toys, they may refrain from talking to their child, and they may use touch and vision to gain attention.

All of these reactions are natural and understandable, but their effect is to distort and impoverish the child's acoustic environment and therefore to impair rather than facilitate auditory development.

linguistic

A child's early linguistic development absolutely depends on conversation with the mother or other caregiver during meaningful interactions —either play or the activities of daily living. When verbal input is withheld or artificially modified (for example, but using only single words), the child's opportunities for language development are reduced.

social and emotional

The most serious effects of parental reaction are felt in the areas of social and emotional development. Children do not need verbal language to sense the fear, anguish, and uncertainty of parents. It is conveyed by their facial expressions, their body odor, and the amount and quality of touching. Their behaviors towards their child become integrated into his or her developing concepts of other people and of self. As the children get older, they may perceive themselves as the cause of their parents' grief. How else are they to interpret the anxiety preceding visits to a clinic at which they are the obvious center of attention and the evident grief afterwards?

While the parents are in a state of guilt-induced impotence, the child is not being provided with appropriate discipline. Limits are not being set because the parents feel helpless, because they are afraid of making mistakes, or because they feel sorry for the child. Unless this problem is resolved, the child will become a tyrant, manipulating the parents mercilessly, testing for limits, and exercising the control which cannot be exercised through language.

It is very difficult for the parents to accept the hearing impairment and any concrete reminders, such as the child's hearing aid. In addition to the practical problems of hearing aid effectiveness, the consequence of this rejection is a further lowering of the child's self-image. The parents may try to be selective—accepting the child while rejecting the hearing loss, but this is impossible. The hearing loss is part of the child. It will remain an important influence on his or her life and personality. The child and the hearing loss cannot be separated. To reject one is to reject the other.

○ VARIATIONS ON A THEME

The foregoing description was that of a child with a profound, congenital, sensorineural hearing loss; no other handicaps; and normally hearing parents. We now consider what happens when some of the significant variables are changed.

moderate hearing loss

The young child with a moderate hearing loss is a more complicated individual than one with a profound loss. Identifying and diagnosing the condition is much more difficult. This child does respond to sound, but inconsistently, and does develop speech and language, but slowly and imperfectly. A basic problem is that the parents, if they are like most of the general public, think of deafness as an all-or-nothing phenomenon. The concept of a partial hearing loss is foreign to them. They are more likely to interpret inconsistent behavior and developmental delay in terms of intellectual or behavioral problems. So too may their pediatrician, unless he or she has an unusually strong grounding in hearing, speech, and language.

When the hearing impairment has been diagnosed and hearing aids fitted, it can still be difficult for the child's parents to understand this condition. They may question the value of amplification, and if it shows no immediate benefit, they may be negligent about its use.

As the child gets older, life can be more frustrating than for a profoundly deaf child. Children with moderate losses follow a normal developmental course, but imperfectly. These youngsters rely on audition, but it frequently lets them down. They communicate verbally but they do not always understand, nor are they always understood. They are like Aesop's fox who sees the grapes and can almost reach them—but not quite.

additional handicaps

When hearing impairment occurs side-by-side with other handicaps, identification and diagnosis can be extremely difficult. Quite simply, the consequences of the hearing impairment are easily masked by or confused with the consequences of the other handicaps. Identification and diagnosis are, therefore, likely to be delayed.

Many of the handicaps that coexist with hearing impairment interact in such a way as to exaggerate its effects on perceptual and linguistic development. The description given in the previous section is still valid, but all the problems are exacerbated.

hearing-impaired parents

When the parents of a profoundly deaf child are themselves deaf, they do not react to the condition in the way I have described. Essentially all of the secondary effects of parental reaction are eliminated. While this may not help the child's auditory or verbal development, it is of immeasurable help to his or her social and emotional development and also to general communicative development.

Teachers of the deaf have known for a long time that the deaf children of deaf parents perform significantly better than the deaf children of hearing parents in every developmental area that is influenced by deafness. It has been suggested that this is due to early use of manual communication by the deaf parents, but research has shown that the effect is still present when the parents do not use sign language. It is reasonable to conclude, then, that the deaf child of deaf parents is at an advantage because the parents are not disabled by the discovery of his or her condition and can more easily provide the security and interaction that are necessary to the development of an emotionally stable, communicatively competent individual.

○ APPROACHES TO HABILITATIVE INTERVENTION

From the foregoing description of development, it will be seen that hearing-impaired children are involved in a kind of chain reaction:

Because of their impairment, they do not learn to hear.

Because they do not learn to hear, they do not acquire language or develop speech.

Because they do not acquire language, their social and emotional development is impaired.

Because they do not develop normally, their parents react in ways that further interfere with all three areas of development.

It follows that early habilitative intervention must address four general issues—hearing, language, social and emotional development, and parental reactions. The relative importance attached to these issues varies according to philosophy and methodology.

emphasis on hearing

The *auditory approach* (also known as *acoupedics* and *the unisensory approach*) is based on the assumption that through early identification and early amplification, it is possible to develop auditory perceptual skills to the point where they can play their natural role in the acquisition of speech and language, thus preventing impairments of communicative, social, and emotional function. The more ardent advocates of this approach do not acknowledge the possibility of a total hearing loss and either state, or imply, that all hearing-impaired children can "learn to hear." In pursuit of this goal they may go so far as to cover their mouths when they talk, in order to prevent lipreading. Those who are less radical acknowledge a ceiling for the auditory performance of individual children but by compensatory measures, try to ensure that this ceiling is reached. Their goal is for hearing to play as great a role as possible in the development of speech and language.

emphasis on speech

For many educators the long term potential of speech as a key to independence and freedom of choice is so compelling that the acquisition of spoken language skills takes top priority, even when this cannot be accomplished through hearing. This philosophy leads to the various oral approaches. Advocates generally believe that the introduction of manual language will interfere with the acquisition of spoken language by removing extrinsic demands. Any delays in the development of linguistic, cognitive, social, or emotional competence that result from strict adherence to this philosophy are considered a small price to pay for the long term benefits.

cued speech

Cued speech provides a system of manual supplements to lipreading with the aim of preserving the benefits of an oral approach while eliminating one of the drawbacks. The hand cues resolve certain ambiguities in the visual speech input and thereby permit full discrimination among speech sounds. Unfortunately, these cues do not provide the sensory feedback needed for establishment of speech competence, nor do they provide input about the prosodic features of speech. Nevertheless, cued speech can accelerate the growth of linguistic and communicative competence for many hearing-impaired children.

emphasis on language and communication

Many educators believe that the most appropriate way to deal with early childhood hearing impairment is by circumvention. What the child needs for cognitive, social, and emotional growth is language. The form in which children acquire language only becomes important if they must interact with people who do not share their language system. This philosophy is expressed in the *Rochester Method* (simultaneous use of speech and finger-spelling) and *Total Communication* (simultaneous use of speech and signs). Proponents argue that mastery of a manual language will serve to enhance the development of spoken language, rather than interfere with it, since the underlying cognitive, linguistic, social, and communicative competencies will be improved.

cognitive emphasis

It is important to remember that language has the same cognitive base, regardless of the modality in which it is expressed. This fact has led some educators, who are disturbed by an excess of concern for form at the expense of substance, to emphasize the need for designing early intervention programs that give the fullest opportunity for development of thinking skills.

parental emphasis

All early intervention programs stress parent involvement, but in many cases the parents are seen mainly as tools for the implementation of specific teaching strategies. Recognition of the fact that the child's development depends on his or her social and emotional well-being, which in turn depends on the emotional well-being of the parents and their feelings and attitudes toward their child, has led to the development of programs in which the primary emphasis is on parent counselling.

emphasis on the child

None of the approaches or methods that evolve from the philosophies just discussed is universally applicable to all hearing-impaired children and their families. To be successful, early intervention must meet three kinds of need:

1. *Basic Needs* that are shared by all children and their families.
2. *Special Needs* that are shared by all hearing-impaired children and their families.
3. *Individual Needs* that are peculiar to the characteristics and circumstances of specific children and their families.

Your responsibility is to identify special and individual needs and address them within the general context of child development and family dynamics. When basic, special, and individual needs come into conflict, you must try to identify the underlying difficulty, discuss it with the parents, and establish a system of goals and priorities that can provide a basis for rational choice. Your greatest allies will be a thorough understanding of the processes involved, readiness to examine your results objectively, and the ability to see the problems from the points of view of the child and the parents.

In the remainder of this book I have tried to define the components of management, to specify objectives, and to suggest ways of reaching them. The tasks of synthesis, adaptation, and establishment of priorities for individual situations must remain yours.

SUMMARY

A severe, profound, or total hearing loss has direct effects on the development of auditory perceptual skills, speech skills, and linguistic skills. The language deficit in turn affects cognitive, social, and emotional development. Following discovery of the hearing impairment, the child's parents enter a period of mourning which includes the reactions of shock, denial, anger, guilt, and passive acceptance. During this period the parents may further undermine their child's development by providing him or her with an impoverished auditory, linguistic, and emotional environment.

Philosophies of intervention place emphasis on different aspects of the problem and lead to various methodological approaches. None of these approaches is uniformly successful with all hearing-impaired children. The responsibility of the teacher is to identify general, special, and individual needs and to adapt procedures accordingly.

FURTHER READING

Helmer Myklebust's text on *The Psychology of Deafness* (Grune & Stratton, New York, 1964) remains one of the most useful sources on the effects of hearing impairment on development, despite the fact that it was first published over twenty years ago. Hilde Schlesinger and Kathryn Meadow's *Sound and Sign* (University of California Press, Berkeley, 1972) focuses mainly on the effects of hearing impairments, and intervention strategies, on mental health. An unusual insight into parental reactions is provided by Susan Gregory in *The Deaf Child and His Family* (John Wiley, New York, 1976), and a multiauthored monograph entitled "The Families of Hearing Impaired Children," edited by A. T. Murphy (*Volta Review,* 81, no. 5, 1979) offers several perspectives on this topic. The mourning process is discussed at length in Elisabeth Kübler-Ross' *On Death and Dying* (Macmillan, New York, 1969).

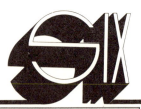

Goals and components of management

The remainder of this book is concerned with practical issues. My aim is to provide a conceptual framework for the organization of a program of early intervention and suggestions for its implementation. I deal first with the child whose sole problem is a severe or profound sensory hearing loss and then discuss the management of children with additional complications. The book ends with a discussion of service delivery and personnel preparation. The present chapter deals with the general goals of intervention and outlines the components of a management program.

○ GOALS OF HABILITATIVE INTERVENTION

long term goals

Why are we intervening in the lives of the hearing-impaired child and his or her family? I suggest it is because we would like the child to develop into an independent adult who is equipped to choose, and to pursue, his or her own road to personal fulfilment. This is, of course, a rather vague and for the infant and preschooler, a very distant objective. Nevertheless, it provides a long term goal against which we can evaluate the validity of more immediate goals.

short term goals

In an early intervention program we prepare the foundation for later development by addressing such goals as

1. Well-adjusted parents with the knowledge and skills to meet their child's needs.
2. A child with a healthy self-image and a desire for social interaction.
3. Reduction of the auditory deficit by proper amplification and auditory training.
4. A child with age-appropriate cognitive skills.
5. A child with language skills that match conceptual development and communicative needs.
6. A child with command of speech as a medium for language.

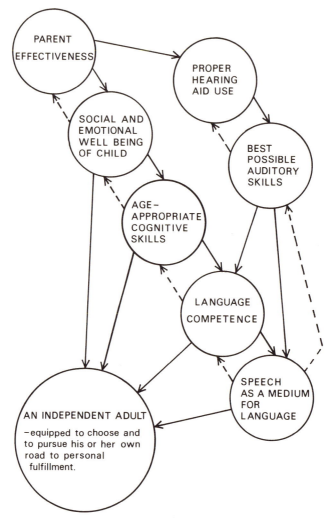

FIGURE 6–1 The Goals of Habilitative Intervention. Short term goals follow a hierarchy in which progress at one level reinforces its own prerequisites (broken lines) as well as preparing the way for realization of subsequent goals (full lines).

With the exception of the third goal (the auditory one), these goals constitute a hierarchy in that a certain amount of success at one level is a prerequisite for progress at the next level. These goals are also, however, mutually dependent. That is to say, attainment of a given goal serves to reinforce its own prerequisites. (See Figure 6–1.) Consider, for example, the relationship between the adjustment of the parents and the language of the child. A secure and stimulating home environment is a prerequisite for healthy emotional and social development which is in turn a prerequisite for language development. Once the child starts to develop language, however, the parents become much more relaxed and are better able to provide a suitable environment. It is as if you are dealing with a plant in which you feed the roots to nurture the leaves which in turn nurture the roots.

Because of their interdependencies, habilitative goals cannot be addressed sequentially. We do not, for example, require the parents to score 80 percent on some behavioral measure before addressing the social and emotional needs of the child, nor do we require high levels of linguistic competence before involving the child in speech-related activities. On the contrary, the short term goals must be addressed simultaneously. Every interaction between you and the parents, or between you and the child, should be designed to facilitate progress towards several goals at once. The hierarchy and the sequence must be in your mind—not in your timetable.

parents' goals

You would do well to explore the question of long and short term goals with the parents. It is quite possible that while you are thinking in terms of maximal auditory development, they are hoping for normal hearing; while you are working for linguistic competence, they are waiting for normal speech; or while you are aiming for independence and self-fulfillment, they are cherishing such goals as "We want him to be like us." Such disparities are counterproductive and should be explored during parent counselling.

priorities

In the ideal situation, the short term intervention goals are mutually compatible. That is to say, the pursuit or attainment of one goal serves to facilitate attainment of all the others. You will, however, encounter situations in which these goals conflict. Consider, for example, the child with advanced communicative needs but negligible competence with spoken language. If you respond to this situation by placing greater emphasis on the mastery of speech to the exclusion of more basic goals, you risk serious and possibly irreversible damage to emotional, social, and cognitive development.

I am touching here on an issue that for many years has polarized the professions serving hearing-impaired children. At one extreme are those educators who believe that command of spoken language is both a necessary and sufficient long term goal that cannot be met if the child learns sign language. At the other extreme are those educators who consider the choice of language modality of secondary importance to the child's immediate need for social, emotional, cognitive, and communicative integrity.

There are, unfortunately, no simple solutions to the problems presented by deafness in early childhood. My advice to you as a teacher is to resist pressures to take sides in the methods controversy and to treat each case on its own merits. You must maintain a clear concept of long and short term goals, relate them to the characteristics and needs of the individual child and the family, and work with the parents to establish priorities.

Rational discussion of this issue is rare because of the deep emotional responses it engenders. You should try, however, to deal with it objectively and to help parents do the same. On a more positive note, let me remind you that one of the benefits to be expected from early intervention is the avoidance of developmental asynchrony with its resulting conflicts of short term goals.

○ COMPONENTS OF MANAGEMENT

The components of habilitative intervention follow naturally from the goals listed earlier. They are

1. *Parental management* including parent counselling, parent education, and parent instruction.
2. *Social and emotional management of the child* to be handled primarily through the parents.
3. *Audiological management* including hearing aid fitting and hearing conservation.
4. *Auditory management* that is, helping the child develop auditory perceptual skills.
5. *Cognitive-linguistic management* that is, helping the child build a detailed and accurate world model and a symbol system to provide access to it.
6. *Speech management* that is, giving the child control of the motor-acoustic symbols of speech and helping him or her learn how to use them linguistically for communication.

Let me stress again that this compartmentalization serves only the needs of organization and exposition. It must not appear in the day-to-day management program. You cannot, for example, treat speech independently of language or hearing independently of speech; you cannot focus on speech and language needs to the exclusion of social and emotional needs; you cannot treat the parents and ignore the child; and you cannot treat the child and ignore the parents. The goals of intervention must be addressed together and in harmony. This kind of synthesis does not come quickly or easily, but once attained it is the mark of a superior teacher.

The six components of habilitative intervention provide the topics for the six chapters which follow, though in a slightly different order from that just presented.

The goals of early habilitative intervention are well-adjusted parents and a child who is emotionally, socially, cognitively, and communicatively competent. Attainment of these goals lays the foundation for further development, leading eventually to an independent adult who is equipped to choose and follow his or her own road to personal fulfillment. In order to meet these goals, intervention must include several components. Though discussed separately for purposes of exposition, these components should be synthesized in a full management program.

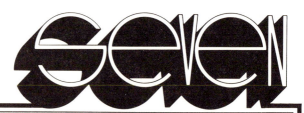

seven

Audiological management

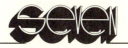

The first responsibility of management is to minimize the hearing impairment. This means, among other things, fitting with hearing aids, developing auditory perceptual skills, and incorporating sound and hearing into general development. In these ways we hope to reduce the severity of the consequences of impairment and to render habilitation simpler and more effective. In the present chapter I discuss those aspects of management designed to deliver acoustic information to the cochlea. The following chapter deals with helping the child to use that information.

○ OBJECTIVES

The objectives of audiological management are as follows:

1. To ensure that the child has appropriate hearing aids.
2. To keep the aids in perfect working order.
3. To establish full time use of the aids.
4. To conserve hearing.
5. To create an optimal acoustic environment.
6. To provide diagnostic information.

The first three objectives apply to children with reduced auditory sensitivity. The second three apply to all hearing-impaired children.

It should be obvious that in this aspect of management teachers and parents must function as members of a team. Since they have the most frequent contact with the child, they are in the best position to provide the kind of reliable and detailed observations on which diagnostic and prescriptive decisions can be made and to identify incipient conductive impairments.

○ PROCEDURES

ensuring that the child is fitted with suitable hearing aids

Because young children do not provide the kind of diagnostic information on which audiologists like to base decisions, hearing aid selection must be viewed as a long term process in which the teacher is an active participant. Initial decisions must be reviewed constantly in the light of response and progress.

The three basic parameters of hearing aid performance are gain, Saturation Sound Pressure Level, and frequency response.

Gain The effect of the hearing aid is to make the child more sensitive to sound. That is to say, the *aided hearing loss* is less than the *unaided hearing loss*. The amount by which the aid reduces the hearing loss is its *gain*. Thus

Hearing Loss – Gain = Aided Hearing Loss

The gain of a hearing aid can be adjusted with the *gain control* (also known as volume control). The appropriate setting is one that enables the child to hear the quieter sounds of conversational speech. To accomplish this we must bring the aided threshold to within 30 dB of the normal threshold of hearing. Thus the appropriate gain equals the unaided hearing loss minus 30 dB. If, for example, a child has a hearing loss of 80 dB, our criterion would be met with a gain of 50 dB, since

80 dB Hearing Loss – 50 dB Gain = 30 dB Aided Hearing Loss

With modern ear level hearing aids and well-made earmolds we can easily provide a 30 dBHL aided threshold for children with moderate and severe hearing losses. If the hearing loss exceeds 90 dB, however, we need gains in excess of 60 dB. This requirement is difficult to meet, not because of the electronics of hearing aids, but because of the problem of acoustic feedback. Attempts to set the gain of an aid to a value greater than about 60 dB usually cause an annoying squeal. Because of this limit we can seldom provide an aided hearing loss as low as 30 dB to profoundly deaf children. If, for example, the loss is 105 dB, we will probably have to be satisfied with an aided threshold of 45 dBHL since

105 dB Hearing Loss – 60 dB Gain = 45 dB Aided Hearing Loss

The teacher has two responsibilities in relation to gain. One is to observe and record the child's responses; the second is to determine the proper setting of the gain control. You should ask whether the child responds to sounds in general and to the quieter speech sounds (such as *m* or *sh*) in particular. The kinds of responses to look for are

cessation of activity in order to listen
searching for the sound source

imitating sounds

vocalizing for pleasure

evidence of sound recognition

correct responses to the *go game*. (See Chapter Eight.)

If a sound level meter is available, use it to measure the quietest levels producing a consistent response. (Note that a level of 30 dBHL corresponds with 40 dBSPL using the *A* setting of a sound level meter.) If responses are obtained to loud sounds but not quiet ones, you should experiment with higher gain control settings. If acoustic feedback prevents you from increasing gain, you must try to deal with this problem by

getting a better earmold (that is, a closer fit, a longer tube, or a denser plastic)

reducing high frequency gain (that is, using the low (L) setting of the tone control or inserting acoustic filters in the mold or sound tubes)

moving the microphone further from the ear (that is, changing from ear level to body aid, or using a CROS fitting. The initials CROS stand for Contralateral Routing Of Signal, an arrangement in which the microphone hangs over one ear while the amplified sound is delivered to the other).

Do not control squealing by turning down the gain unless *all other possibilities* have been exhausted.

You should note that gain settings can be too high as well as too low. Increasing the gain beyond the value giving a 30 dB aided hearing loss causes excessive amplification of background noise and reverberation and may, at the same time, clip and distort the louder sounds of speech. This makes it harder for the child to differentiate speech from noise or to discriminate among speech sounds. Only for children with mild or moderate losses and wide dynamic ranges are aided thresholds of less than 30 dBHL appropriate.

Before leaving the topic of gain, I must make one more point. Laboratory tests of a hearing aid do not give exact information about how it will perform on a child's ear. The actual gain depends not only on the aid but also on the acoustic properties of the earmold and the ear and on the fit between earmold and ear. Optimal setting of the gain control cannot, therefore, be determined solely from electroacoustic measurements. The ultimate criterion for the correctness of gain setting is the performance of the child while wearing the aid. Hence the importance of teacher observation.

Saturation Sound Pressure Level (SSPL)   The *Saturation Sound Pressure Level* of an aid (also called the maximum power output) is the strongest sound it is capable of delivering. Sounds are prevented from exceeding this level by a process called *peak clipping* or in some cases by special *compression* circuitry. Peak clipping is simple and inexpensive but causes distortion of the clipped signal. Compression causes less distortion but is more complicated.

The sound level entering the child's ear is the sum of the sound level entering the microphone and the gain of the aid. Thus

$$\text{Input} + \text{Gain} = \text{Output}$$

If, however, the sum of input and gain exceeds the SSPL, this simple equation no longer applies. Instead, we have

$$\text{Input} + \text{Gain} = \text{SSPL} + \text{Distortion}$$

Selection and adjustment of SSPL are based on two criteria:

1. The need to provide an adequate dynamic range between the threshold of hearing and the SSPL of the aid. Ideally, this range should be at least 30 dB to provide audibility of the quieter sounds of speech without distorting the louder sounds.

2. The need to avoid discomfort to the child or the risk of further damage to the delicate mechanisms within the cochlea.

These two criteria are sometimes incompatible, in which case the second must take priority.

What are the teacher's responsibilities in relation to SSPL? Exactly the same as with gain—observation and adjustment. Observe and record any signs of pain or discomfort to loud sounds. Examples are

startle reflexes
eye blinks
involuntary head jerks
crying
repeated removal of aid
refusal to wear aid.

If these responses are observed, you must remember that excessive power is only one possible reason. Hearing-impaired children need to get used to sound, and their tolerance for amplification improves with experience.

Adjustment of SSPL is possible on some, but not all, hearing aids. (See Figure 7–1). If the child is showing signs of discomfort, the power should be reduced. If this does not solve the problem, you should look for other causes, such as uncomfortable earmolds or manipulative behavior.

Please note that the problem of excessive SSPL cannot be solved by reducing the gain of the aid. Turning down the volume control may bring conversational speech to a comfortable level, but the child will still be disturbed by loud inputs, such as shouting and banging, and the chances are that the quieter speech sounds will be rendered inaudible. The rule is:

> Increase the gain to the point where the quieter speech sounds become audible and reduce the SSPL so that the aid is incapable of generating an uncomfortably loud sound.

If the child's dynamic range, from threshold of audibility to threshold of discomfort, is less than 20 or 30 dB, it may be necessary to try aids that compress the intensity range of speech.

FIGURE 7–1   Adjusting the Saturation Sound Pressure Level of a behind-the-ear hearing aid.

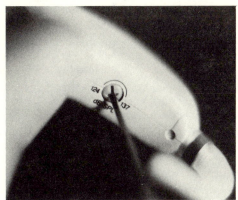

FIGURE 7–2   Adjusting the frequency response of a behind-the-ear hearing aid.

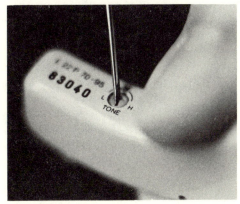

The comments I made earlier about the difference between laboratory tests and real ear performance apply to SSPL, just as they do to gain.

Frequency Response Hearing aids typically have different gains at different frequencies. The relationship between gain and frequency is referred to as the *frequency response.* When we adjust the tone control of a hearing aid, we modify the frequency response, emphasizing high frequencies at the expense of low frequencies, or vice versa.

Selection of frequency response is based on several criteria:

1. A desire for high fidelity. This would involve equal gain at all frequencies, otherwise known as a *flat response.*
2. A desire to amplify speech at the expense of ambient noise. This involves a suppression of the low frequencies that contain most of the energy in environmental noise.
3. A desire to prevent the masking of high frequencies by low frequencies. We reduce the masking effect by emphasizing high frequencies at the expense of low frequencies.
4. A desire to provide maximum amplification in those frequencies to which the child is most sensitive. For the majority of profoundly deaf children this criterion calls for emphasis of the low frequencies.
5. A desire to avoid excessive acoustic feedback. The effects of acoustic feedback are most pronounced at high frequencies. To reduce feedback we must, therefore, reduce high frequency gain.

Control of frequency response is accomplished with a tone control. Such controls typically have a normal (N) position that involves moderate high frequency emphasis, a low (L) position that reduces the high frequency gain and a high (H) position that reduces the low frequency gain. (See Figure 7–2.) As a rule of thumb, children with moderate and severe losses should use either the N or H positions to provide the best separation of speech from noise and the greatest clarity of the speech. Profoundly deaf children, with only low frequency hearing, often benefit from the L position, since this setting emphasizes the low frequencies while reducing the effects of acoustic feedback. You should note, however, that as with gain and SSPL, the performance of an aid on a child's ear is highly dependent on the characteristics of the earmold, the acoustical properties of the ear, and the fit of earmold to ear. Once again, therefore, it becomes the responsibility of the teacher to observe responses, especially in a noisy environment, and perhaps to experiment with changes of frequency response.

Let me repeat that the teacher's role in relation to hearing aids is as part of a team. All observations of behavior and any changes in hearing aid characteristics, together with information on the child's progress, must be communicated to and discussed with the audiologist responsible for selecting the aids.

keeping the hearing aids in perfect working order

The nature of hearing aids and the conditions under which they must be used make the probability of equipment failure extremely high. It is, therefore, imperative that the status and performance of a young child's hearing aid be checked at least daily and that immediate repair or replacement be effected if a problem is found. Hearing aids can be checked by eye, by ear, by finger, and by instrument.

By eye Examine the aid for signs of physical damage such as

Cracks in the case, the receiver, the tubing, or the earmold.

Loose connections between the aid and the tubing, between cord sockets and plugs, between different sections of tubing, or between receiver and earmold.

Frayed cords.

Dirt in the microphone inlet, the tubing, or the earmold.

Corroded battery contacts.

By ear Turn the hearing aid on and make sure that it squeals when the gain control is turned up. Then listen to the sound coming out of the hearing aid as you talk into it. For this purpose you should use a listening stethoscope as shown in Figure 7–3. Listening with a stethoscope permits you

To listen with both ears.

To listen at more comfortable levels than if you were to use an earmold.

To check the whole system, including the child's earmold.

You should be listening for

Weak output, or no output at all.

Distorted output (for example, tinny, muffled, or raspy sound).

Extraneous hissing and buzzing noises or intermittent crackling sounds as you manipulate the gain control, operate the switches, and flex the cords.

A common complaint of teachers and parents is, "I don't know what to listen for—it always sounds distorted to me." There is no way to tell you in print about the quality of normal and defective amplification. You must train yourself to hear these characteristics. The mistake many teachers make is to

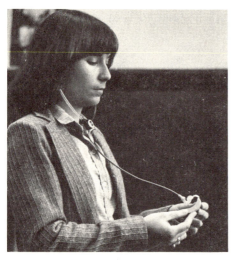

FIGURE 7-3 Using a listening stethoscope to check a hearing aid "by ear." Parents must be taught to listen to their child's aid at least once a day.

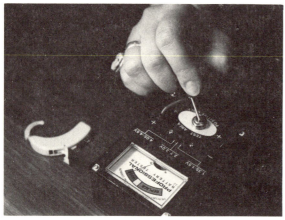

FIGURE 7-4 An inexpensive battery tester can be used to check the condition of hearing aid batteries.

listen to aids only when they think there is a fault. By listening to them regularly on a routine, daily basis, you will accumulate the kind of experience needed to detect faults when they do occur.

Make sure that you listen to all amplification channels when checking hearing aids. If a child has two receivers, listen to both. If he or she is wearing a group hearing aid or a wireless system, listen using both student microphone and teacher microphone.

Make sure that you check the whole system from microphone to earmold. Earmolds easily become blocked with wax and with water left from improper drying. You must listen to the sound coming *out* of the earmold, not just the sound entering it.

By finger I mentioned earlier that the gain of a hearing is limited by the problem of acoustic feedback. It is extremely important that the output of the hearing aid be prevented from reaching the microphone, otherwise the aid simply amplifies its own output, and squealing results. One cause of excessive acoustic feedback is a poor fit between earmold and ear. A poor fit is not the only cause, however. Sound can leak out through the walls of the earmold; through cracks in the earmold, sound tube, or receiver; and through connections between various parts of the aid. It can also leak inside the aid because of broken or displaced parts. To check for acoustic feedback, simply place your finger over the sound outlet from the earmold, and turn the gain control to its highest value. If all is well, the aid will not squeal (though it should do so immediately if you remove your finger). If the aid does squeal, you can try to track down the problem by removing the mold and testing again. With ear level aids you can also remove the ear hook and check for internal feedback.

By instrument You can make sure that the battery is still functional by checking its voltage with a simple battery tester. (See Figure 7–4.) If you are more abitious, you can measure the decibel output of the aid, and its maximum power output, using a sound level meter and an acoustic coupler. (See Figure 7–5.) At least one manufacturer of group amplification equipment provides measuring instruments that are built into the charging unit. These provide information on gain, maximum output, and the condition of receiver and connecting cords. The most ambitious step is to purchase a hearing aid test box that provides measurements of gain, maximum power output, frequency response, and distortion. (See Figure 7–6.) Purchase of expensive test equipment only makes sense when there are several children to be handled, and even then it may be better to contract for hearing aid test services with an audiology center. As a rule of thumb, you should arrange for full electroacoustic evaluation of a young child's hearing aid once a month.

When a fault is detected in the hearing aid, it should obviously be remedied. There are some procedures that teachers and parents can learn to carry out for themselves. Batteries, cords, receivers, and sound tubing can be replaced; battery contacts can be cleaned with a pencil eraser; cracked cases can be taped up; and dirt can be removed from earmolds. Repair problems you cannot handle yourself must be passed on to a hearing aid technician, a hearing aid dealer, or a repair center. If there is to be a delay in returning the aid, a backup aid should be provided for the child. *This loaner must be of the same type as the child's own aid and should be adjusted in the same way.* It is not appropriate to look through a box of discarded aids to find one that works. Some parents purchase a spare aid so that their child will have his or her own backup. As a practical goal, a child should not be without a hearing aid for more than 24 hours in any one month.

Before leaving the topic of hearing aid monitoring, I should say a little more about earmolds. These seemingly insignificant pieces of rubber or

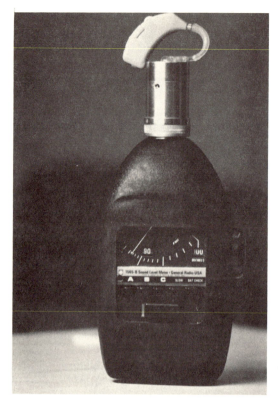

FIGURE 7-5 With a sound level meter and a simple coupler, you can estimate the gain and SSPL of a hearing aid using speech as the input.

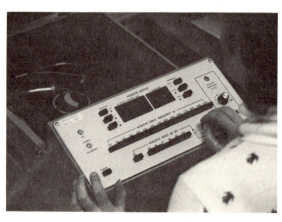

FIGURE 7-6 The Hearing Aid Test Box is relatively easy to use and provides exact information on gain, SSPL, frequency response, and distortion.

plastic are one of the most critical parts of an aid. As I mentioned earlier, the aid's performance is dependent on the acoustic properties of the mold and on the way it fits the ear. A leaky earmold causes feedback problems, reduces available gain, and severely diminishes low frequency response. You should, however, avoid the temptation to get molds that are oversize

—fitting the ear canal like a cork. Living tissue resists pressure by modifying its shape. The long term effect of oversized earmolds is an enlarged ear canal.

In addition to ensuring that the mold is accurate and of the highest quality, weekly cleaning is essential. The mold should be washed in warm, soapy water, rinsed in clean water, and *thoroughly dried* before being replaced on the aid. A drop of water in the earmold reduces output and gain by 30 or 40 dB. The most efficient way of drying the mold is to use a blower, as shown in Figure 7–7.

establishing full-time use of the aids

Children who are using hearing aids successfully accept them as part of themselves—as an extension of their hearing mechanisms. They do not listen to the sounds coming out of the aids but to the sounds entering them. The microphones become their ears, and they are uncomfortable and disoriented when the aids do not work. How do we reach this desirable state of affairs?

The first step is parent counselling. If parents do not accept the aids, neither will their child. But acceptance is difficult for them. The hearing aids serve as a concrete reminder of the hearing impairment. Stern lectures on the importance of the aids and attempts to make the parents feel guilty when the aids are not worn are not useful approaches to the problem. Your responsibility is to facilitate constructive acceptance and to act as a sounding board, freely acknowledging and discussing any negative feelings about the hearing aids. Also, be careful not to mislead the parents into believing that the hearing aids will be a cure for the deafness and that they will eliminate

FIGURE 7–7 An air blower should be used to dry the inside of the newly washed earmold before replacement on the hearing aid.

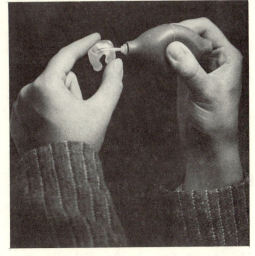

the hearing problem. Such misinformation only prolongs the denial stage of mourning. (See also the chapter on parent management.)

Step two is to establish the routine wearing of the aids. Putting on the aids must become as automatic as getting dressed. Parents should know that except for swimming and for a few other potentially harmful activities, the aids must remain in place until bed time, and perhaps even be left in place until the child is asleep.

If the child resists the hearing aids, your first responsibility is to determine the cause. Possibilities are

1. Uncomfortable earmolds.
2. Excessive Saturation Sound Pressure Level.
3. The annoyance of unaccustomed sound.
4. General negativism aggravated by the parents' ambivalence and nervousness in relation to the aids.

The first two problems should be dealt with by changing the earmolds and reducing the maximum power output respectively. The other two are less easily resolved. It is very common for a child who is more than eighteen months old to reject hearing aids simply because the sounds they generate are intrusive. Perceptually and cognitively this child has been developing very nicely without audition and the noises from the aid are disturbing. To avoid rejection, you must introduce the child to the world of sound gradually. This means increasing the gain a little day by day, starting with a low, but tolerable, value. It also means increasing the length of time during which the aids are worn. In the beginning, the wearing of the aids can be associated with a particularly pleasant activity. It is best to choose a quiet time when the child can have his or her mother's undivided attention and the two can play with a favorite toy or do something that is mutually satisfying, such as looking at books. It is also important that the activity involve meaningful use of sounds, some of which are generated by the child. Playing with noise-making toys, and conversation, meet this criterion—watching television does not. If the child is an ardent TV watcher, however, viewing time can be used to advantage as an *additional* time during which wearing of the aid is required.

A frequent problem with young hearing-impaired children is that the hearing aids become a pawn in the conflict over independence and control that typically begins between the second and third birthdays. If this is not to stand in the way of effective auditory development, it is essential that the parents resolve their own inner conflicts about the aids and that they understand the child's needs for discipline and limits—a need that is just as great as that of the hearing child's, (perhaps even greater since predictability and consistency must in part substitute for language; see Chapter Nine). You must provide the parents with support as they adapt to the problems of parenting a child with special needs.

The next step to ensuring full time hearing aid use is to make sound meaningful. Audition must be something that works for children—getting them what they want, and facilitating interactions with their environment. All of the work on auditory development, hearing aid maintenance, and hearing conservation that is discussed elsewhere in this chapter and in the next chapter contribute to the goal of full time hearing aid use.

conserving hearing

There are three major ways in which a child's hearing can deteriorate:

1. Spontaneous cochlear degeneration.
2. Cochlear damage resulting from drugs, disease, trauma, or excessive noise.
3. Development of conductive disorders, such as a blocked ear canal or inflammation of the middle ear.

At best, hearing-impaired children are as susceptible as other children to further loss of hearing. At worst, they are more susceptible by virtue of genetic weakness, existing cochlear deficiencies, and the need for constant exposure to very loud sounds. The teacher's responsibilities are prevention, identification, and referral.

Prevention You can reduce the likelihood of further cochlear damage by

1. Avoiding the use of higher hearing aid outputs than are absolutely necessary.
2. Encouraging good nutrition and general hygiene.
3. Ensuring that parents seek prompt medical attention for any illnesses involving fever.
4. Ensuring immediate audiological and otological evaluation following severe head blows.

You can help to prevent blockage of ear canals by

1. Encouraging parents to clean the *entrance* (but *only* the entrance) to the ear canal regularly. (Note that the earmold interferes with the body's natural ear-cleaning mechanism.)
2. Establishing routine ear examinations by a physician (minimum of once every three to six months).

You can help to reduce the duration of middle ear disorders and minimize the likelihood of permanent damage by

1. Teaching parents how to recognize the signs of incipient otitis media (see the
   following section).
2. Ensuring that immediate medical evaluation and treatment are sought if an ear
   infection develops.

Identification Make sure that hearing status is reviewed regularly.
Young hearing-impaired children should have their hearing tested once
every three months and this testing should include *tympanometry.* Tympanometry involves measuring the sound reflecting properties of the tympanic membrane and the way in which these properties change as the
pressure in the ear canal is varied. It is a simple, speedy procedure and is
a very powerful aid in the identification and diagnosis of middle ear disorders. Children who are known to be subject to recurring ear infections
should receive routine tympanometry once a month.

Learn to use an otoscope, and examine the child's ear canals routinely
once a week. Look for an excessive accumulation of wax or debris.

Learn the signs of incipient otitis media. These are

1. Reduction of auditory responsiveness—child no longer turns when called or
   fails to respond to familiar sounds.
2. Pain and discomfort around the ear—not always a reliable indicator. After
   several ear infections, a child may no longer experience pain with this condition.
3. Unaccustomed feedback problems with aid—sometimes the first sign of a
   conductive problem is that a previously well-behaved aid begins to squeal.
   You will recall that the gain and output of a hearing aid depend partly on the
   acoustic properties of the ear. One consequence of a blocked ear canal or
   a fluid-filled middle ear is an increase in the sound reflected from the tympanic
   membrane. This increases acoustic feedback, thus causing the aid to squeal.

Referral Ensure that any confirmed or suspected changes of hearing status are referred for audiological and otological evaluation. If you are
dealing with spontaneous degeneration, the sooner it is recognized, the
sooner the child's program of management can be modified. If you are
dealing with a reversible change, early referral should reduce its duration
and also the possibility of irreversible damage.

creating an optimal acoustic environment

The ideal acoustic environment for children who are learning to use
their defective hearing has a maximum of meaningful sound and a minimum
of interfering noise. Of course, the distinction between the two is not easily

defined. The continuous sound of television may provide companionship to a lonely mother but is interfering noise to her hearing-impaired child. Children on the other hand, find great meaning in the sound they can make with a tin can and a block, while the same sound may drive their parents to distraction.

The general principles should be   .

1. Eliminate unnecessary sounds and sounds that have no relevance to the child.
2. Provide the child with lots of sound that is inherently meaningful.
3. Give the child experience of sounds so that as many sounds as possible are upgraded from the *interfering noise* category to the *meaningful sound* category.

Examples of unnecessary sounds are

TVs and radios that play continuously when no one is watching or listening.

Certain aquarium pumps.

Rattling saucepans when they are used repeatedly by parents to "test" their child's hearing.

Impact noise from bare floors and reverberation from bare walls and ceilings.

Examples of sounds that can become meaningful are

Door chimes.

The garage door opening when a parent comes home.

The sounds of food preparation.

The sound of TV when it signals the start of a favorite program.

Any sounds created by the child.

The sounds of human speech when it is addressed to the child or when it signals the presence of a particular person.

In certain learning situations an extremely favorable speech-to-noise ratio can be obtained with auditory training units—either the wired or the wireless variety. The significant feature of these devices is that the microphone is close to the source of speech which is therefore picked up at a high decibel level. For the very young child, however, auditory training systems must be used with extreme caution, if they are used at all. They create a very unnatural situation in which the child's "new ear" (that is, the microphone) is some distance from his or her head. This is liable to interfere with the development of auditory perceptual skills, especially those relating to attention and the auditory perception of space. (See Chapter Eight.)

providing diagnostic information

One of the teacher's responsibilities is to make careful observations that will help to confirm, contradict, or refine initial evaluative or prescriptive decisions. You should note and report any information of relevance to

location of damage to the auditory mechanism

degree of hearing loss

presence of additional problems that may influence learning

suitable amplification

Let me reiterate that the teacher, as the professional having the most direct contact with the child, is a critical member of the audiological-otological management team. Teachers, in turn, must educate parents, who have still more direct contact, so that they too will provide reliable and meaningful information about their children.

○ EVALUATION

Keep careful records of hearing aid settings, the results of electroacoustic evaluation, the results of daily checks, and the incidence of breakdowns. Until the aids are in full time use, have parents keep records of the amount of time for which they are worn. Maintain cumulative audiological records, with information on aided and unaided threshold. From information of this type, you should be able to report on how well the objectives listed at the beginning of this chapter are being met. (See also Appendix A and Appendix B.)

If we are to take full advantage of limited hearing ability, we must deliver the best possible acoustic signals to the child's cochlea. In collaboration with other members of the audiological management team, the teacher can ensure that hearing aid gain is sufficient to bring the quieter sounds of speech to a level of audibility

that Saturation Sound Pressure Level is high enough to accommodate the intensity range of speech but not so high as to cause pain or cochlear damage

that the frequency response of the aids provides a clear speech signal without excessive ambient noise

that the aids remain in perfect working order and in full time use

that the child's auditory sensitivity does not get worse

that the acoustic environment is such as to provide a maximum of meaningful sound with a miminum of interfering noise

that detailed and reliable information is collected on the child's audiological status, responses to amplification, and progress in auditory development.

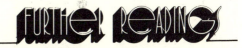

The chapter entitled "Hearing Aids for Children" in Jerry Northern and Marion Downs' book *Hearing in Children*—second edition (Williams & Wilkins, Baltimore, Md., 1978) provides a nice balance between literature review and practical suggestions.

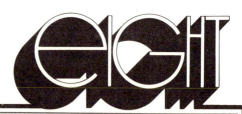

EIGHT

Auditory management

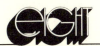

The immediate purpose of auditory management is to help the hearing-impaired child learn how to hear. Children with severe or profound hearing losses, wearing hearing aids for the first time, do not know how to interpret the neural patterns generated by their cochleas. To the extent that we can control our interactions with them and their interactions with the environment, we must try to create situations that will stimulate and reward auditory learning. Eventually, we hope to use auditory skills to increase the rate and quality of social and communicative development.

○ OBJECTIVES

If auditory management is successful, the hearing-impaired child will

1. Attend to sounds.
2. Attend to differences among sounds.
3. Recognize objects and events from the sounds they make.
4. Be alerted by sounds.
5. Use hearing for the perception of space.
6. Use hearing for the perception of speech.
7. Use hearing to control the production of speech.

You will note that these objectives are qualitative, not quantitative. Objective 3, for example, states only that the child will recognize objects and events by means of sound but does not state what kind, how many, or how accurately. Thus, within each general objective, there is room for the delineation of many specific objectives in the programs of individual children.

○ SKILL DEVELOPMENT

As you plan your interactions with the child, either directly, in tutoring or classroom situations, or indirectly, by means of parent education and counselling, you should be thinking, among other things, of ways to realize the objectives just listed. At the same time, you must keep in mind that there are five requirements for the establishment of a skill—physiological capacity, subskills (or readiness skills), motivation, reward, and generalization.

capacity

It must be physiologically possible for the child to acquire the skill. You should not, for example, expect a child with no hearing to recognize sounds, any more than you would expect a child with no arms to do handstands. In practice, you may not be justified in assuming absence of the capacity until all your best efforts at establishing the skill have failed. Nevertheless, the concept of capacity is very important to planning and evaluation.

subskills

Before expecting a child to acquire new skills, you must be sure that he or she has mastered any critical subskills. It is not always possible to know which subskills are essential or whether they have been mastered, but as with capacity, the concept of a hierarchy of subskills is important. If a child is having difficulty with a particular task, you should consider the possibility of working on something more basic.

motivation

As you structure the child's physical and social environment, you must create an extrinsic need for the acquisition of new skills. This may involve the capitalization on the child's intrinsic needs for such things as exploration, communication, and approval. Take care, however! If you truly create a need for a skill for which the capacity or subskills are lacking, the child will be frustrated, and you will do more harm than good. It is because of the dangers of overchallenging that the concepts of capacity and subskills are so important.

reward

If children are to develop auditory skills, it must be worth the effort. Hearing must gain them benefits they cannot gain in any other way. Eventually, you hope these benefits will be derived from the mastery of verbal communication skills. At first, however, you will have to think in more basic terms. See to it that audition satisfies the children's need to know what is going on around them. Let them discover that sound can control people. Let sound be their first clue to the presence of things they want and enjoy.

practice

Once a skill has been acquired, you must provide countless opportunities for its rehearsal and generalization. It must soak into the fabric of the child's existence. Just because you can honestly report that you have met one of the objectives listed earlier, you are not justified in forgetting about it. You must expand and consolidate on the new skill, until it can be sustained by the child's natural environment.

○ PROCEDURES

In this section I suggest ways of helping the hearing-impaired child reach each of the objectives listed earlier. Please do not interpret the following as a curriculum or a "method." Accept it merely as a starting point from which to develop the auditory component of intervention programs for the real children whose management you undertake.

developing attention to sound   *2/08 76*

When first fitted with hearing aids, hearing-impaired children are likely to be distracted by the noises they hear. Since these children are unable to interpret the noises, they will quickly reject them—either by rejecting the aids or by ignoring the sounds. You must redirect their attention and show them that sound carries meaning. There are at least three situations in which you can do this.

If, for example, you are interacting with a child and you hear an unexpected sound, stop what you are doing, look around, look puzzled, possibly raise your hand to your ear, and tell the child you heard something. Then smile with recognition, tell the child what you heard, and take him or her to see the source. Examples might be a dog barking outside, a carpenter working in another room, or an airplane flying overhead. Do not limit yourself to the more obvious, loud, or disturbing sounds. Train yourself to become aware of the quieter sounds of everyday life, such as the toilet flushing or the rain hitting the window. Remember that you must act as the child's "auditory watchdog" until his or her own skills are sufficiently developed.

In the foregoing situation, the sound was an intrusion, and you gave it meaning by taking the child to see the source. It frequently happens, however, that sound occurs as an integral part of the child's activity. In such cases you can draw attention to the sound by dissociating it from other aspects of sensation—for example by turning the child around and making the sound out of his or her line of sight. Suppose that the two of you are playing with a bus and you notice the sound made when the child spins the wheels. Take the bus, spin the wheels, hold the bus to your ear in obvious delight, tell the child you hear the bus, exhort him or her to listen, spin the wheels again, and hold the bus to the child's ear.

The third situation involves the use of sound as the key component of a game—what we might call the *go game*. Engage the child in some repeated activity, such as building a tower, switching the light off and on, or eating cereal. Establish a game in which the word *go* is the signal for each repetition. Allow the child to see and hear you until the rules are clearly understood. Then dissociate the auditory sensation by moving out of the line of sight. (Note that any sound can be substituted for the word *go*.) In this last activity you must be prepared to change roles with the child. In addition to maintaining motivation, this teaches the child that other people can be controlled by sound. Take care that the child does not just respond randomly. Take care, also, not to give the impression that you are testing. This identical activity will be used in audiological testing, but it loses its value as an auditory learning experience unless it remains a game in the child's mind.

The three examples just cited may be summarized as follows:

> Draw attention to unexpected sounds by reacting yourself, and give them meaning by associating them with visual experiences.
>
> Draw attention to sounds that result from the child's own activities by dissociating them from other aspects of experience.
>
> Draw attention to anticipated sounds by making the child's response contingent on them.

developing attention to differences among sounds

In the three situations just described, the child's task was to ask and answer the question, "Was there a sound?" If we wish to draw attention to differences among sounds, we must present two or more and require him or her to answer the question, "Which sound did you hear?" This kind of activity may be referred to as a *multiple choice* or *discrimination* task.

Suppose, for example, you are playing with two or three toys, each of which makes a different sound. Establish a game in which the child imitates your actions, making whichever sound you just made. When the task is understood, turn the child around and require decisions on the basis of hearing alone. As soon as possible, increase the number of options.

I must stress that this activity does not require recognition. The child is not answering, "What did you hear?" but "Which did you hear?" This is not a trivial semantic distinction. In fact, the difference is so important that you should avoid multiple choice tasks if at all possible. Use them as a stepping stone to true recognition, or as a way of collecting diagnostic information, but keep them to a minimum. The problem is that with practice in this kind of activity, children can learn to get the right answer for the wrong reasons. They may learn, for example, that the louder sound is the crying doll and the quieter sound is the musical apple—or worse, that if they hear a sound, it is the drum and if they hear nothing, it must have been the bell. This process is entirely different from recognition which involves learning to abstract from complex sounds those features which are invariant. Loudness, for example, is seldom a critical feature for recognition since we must be able to recognize sounds at varying distances. In multiple choice tasks, however, loudness can easily become the most important response criterion.

Another problem with multiple choice tasks is the high probability of correct guessing. If there are only two alternatives, for example, there is obviously a 50 percent probability that the child will guess correctly. To be certain that correct responses are not chance happenings, you must keep repeating the activity—perhaps to the point of boredom. In fact, you need at least five consecutive correct responses before you can feel reasonably confident of performance. (With three or four alternatives, this reduces to three consecutive correct responses, and with five or more alternatives, two consecutive correct responses are sufficient.)

There is a place for multiple choice activities in auditory work with certain hearing-impaired children, but remember that they have a specific goal—to draw attention to differences among sounds. Do not overdo it.

developing auditory recognition skills

The essential difference between multiple choice activities and true recognition lies in the *location* of the response options. When you ask "Which did you hear?" the response options are defined by you and are external to the child. When you ask, "What did you hear?" the response options are defined by and are internal to, the child. The options become the categories into which the child has organized the world model we discussed in Chapter Three. If the answer is externalized, this will be done by imitation, mime, gesture, or symbol.

To help children develop auditory recognition skills, you must provide them with multiple opportunities to discover the associations between sound sensations and the other modalities by which they have already developed their perceptual world. These modalities are motoric, tactile, and visual.

Activities in which the child is the generator of sound offer the most effective kinds of association. (See Figure 8–1.) Banging a spoon on a plate, shaking a rattle, or kicking the side of a crib, involve moving, feeling, seeing, and hearing all at the same time. In the special case of speech sounds, the visual component is missing, but the child can still associate movement, touch and hearing.

For those sounds which the child cannot make, we must be satisfied with auditory-visual association. That is to say, we make sure the child sees the sound being made. (See Figure 8–2.) Whatever the level of association, we must also try to encourage attention to sound by dissociation as described earlier.

A word of caution—teachers sometimes use auditory-pictorial association for auditory training. That is to say, they show the child a picture of the object that makes the sound being heard. This may be useful for the auditorily advanced child but is useless as an introduction to the world of sound. In a sense it is dishonest. The picture is not making the sound but merely serves as a nonverbal symbol for the true source. The same reservation must be applied to auditory-verbal association. It is not enough to say, "Listen. I hear a truck." If it is the child's first experience of this sound, you must take him or her to see its source.

So far I have discussed the prerequisites for the development of auditory recognition—attention and association. Now we must consider how we help children discover that they can decide "What made the sound" on the basis of hearing alone. One possibility is to ask them the question. Consider, for example, the situation discussed earlier in which you draw the child's attention to an intrusive sound. After you say, "I heard something," follow it with, "Yes! You heard something—what did you hear?" If the child cannot answer promptly, give the answer, and then continue as before. The important thing is that you draw attention to the sound and then give the opportunity to make decisions about it.

Another example involves the use of noise-making objects. Put a selection of them into a brown paper bag, and let the child guess what you are going to bring out by listening to its noise. If he or she guesses wrongly, do not push the issue, simply bring out the object, and go through the association-dissociation routine discussed earlier.

Yet another way of promoting auditory decision making is to take every opportunity of using sound as the child's first source of information about a significant (to him or her) object or event. If you are about to walk into the child's room, for example, talk loudly so you can be heard before you are seen. If it is time for a favorite TV program, switch the set on so that the sound can be heard first. In a sense, this is Pavlovian conditioning. The child first hears the sound and then becomes aware of what is making it. After a sufficient number of exposures, he or she will become aware of what is making it as soon as it is heard.

Recognition is at the core of auditory development. Your major effort should be devoted to developing the subskills and exercising the process. As you do this, you must remember that recognition skills develop from *repeated exposure* to sound patterns and *experience of the full range of permissible variations* in those patterns. The child's task is to abstract, from multiple examples, those features of the sound pattern which are consistent, and

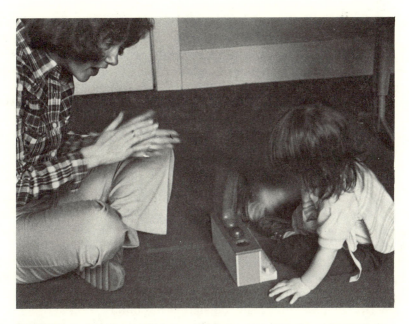

FIGURE 8–1 Activities in which the child is the generator of sound provide the opportunity for association of auditory, motor, tactile, and visual sensations and thereby promote the development of auditory recognition skills.

FIGURE 8–2 When watching someone, or something, else generate sound, the child is restricted to auditory-visual association for facilitation of the development of auditory recognition skills.

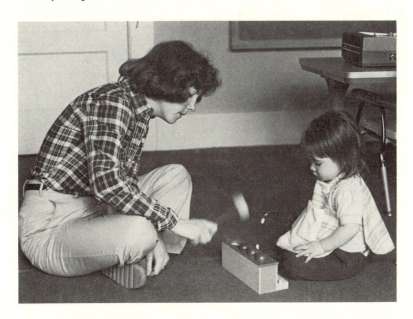

therefore informative, and to ignore those features which are inconsistent and therefore uninformative. This cannot be accomplished with either a single exposure to a sound or repeated exposure to an identical sound (such as might be provided by a tape or phonograph recording). If auditory recognition is to develop, you must fill the child's day with varied examples of meaningful sounds that can be associated with motoric, visual, and tactile experiences, and you must engage the child in activities that draw attention to sound and require decisions to be made about its source.

using sound to gain the child's attention

You can help to make hearing worthwhile for children by using sound to get their attention prior to a change of activity. The most obvious example is to call them by name. If they do not respond within three calls, go and get their attention visually, but tell them that you called, go through the association-dissociation routine, and then continue with what you were doing. It is important that you be relaxed and casual about this. Do not convey a sense of frustration at the children's failure to respond. If they have the capacity, they will eventually be alerted by sound.

Do not limit yourself to name calling. When it is time to eat, make conspicuous noises with the crockery. When it is time for bathing, start filling the tub. When the doorbell rings, give the child a chance to be the first to respond. You will note that these activities are similar to the conditioning process discussed at the end of the previous section. There is a difference, however. You are now creating a waiting time during which the child has an opportunity to attend to, and make decisions about, the sound. There will, of course, be occasions on which the child chooses not to do this. He or she is then exercising a right enjoyed by every normally hearing child.

This deceptively simple activity represents a synthesis of auditory skills. It requires detection, attention, discrimination, recognition, comprehension, and involves the meaningful use of sound. A word of caution is necessary, however. You must only get the child's attention when there is a good reason. Alerting activities must be a precursor to something relevant and meaningful. Calling children's names, just to see if they will respond, is counterproductive. They quickly discover that there is nothing in it for them and they learn to ignore you. For this reason you must encourage parents to refrain from continually "testing" by name calling, pan banging, and so on. Keep in mind that our goal is to make sound and hearing work for the child—not for ourselves.

developing the auditory perception of space

You do not need to do anything special about auditory space perception. All of the child's listening experiences, especially those requiring the meaningful use of sound, will help to answer the question, "Where did the sound come from?"

In the beginning, sound will be a sensation, perceived in the ear and apparently originating from the hearing aid. As children discover the true sources of sound, however, they will externalize their auditory sensations and will perceive them at their point of origin. The sound of the telephone will seem to come from the telephone—the sound of your speech will seem to come from your mouth—and so on. We are all familiar with this phenomenon if we have ever watched a movie. The speech sounds seem to come from the mouths of the actors even though the loudspeakers may be located elsewhere.

The phenomenon just described involves fitting auditory sensations into an already established knowledge of space. We perceive the sound at its source only because we know where its source is. There is, however, another aspect to auditory space perception that can function independently of other perceptual modalities—directional hearing. This is the ability to interpret time and intensity differences between the sound patterns arriving at the two ears in terms of a direction of origin. This phenomenon makes it possible for us to answer, "Where did the sound come from?" *before* we answer, "What made the sound?"

Many hearing-impaired children can develop directional hearing skills, but only if they have compatible auditory capacities in the two ears and if they wear two separate hearing aids. There is much anecdotal evidence to suggest that the development of true directional hearing accelerates auditory development by improving alerting and attentional behaviors and helping the child to separate meaningful sound patterns from a background of noise.

Note again that to take advantage of the capacity for directional hearing, if it exists, we must use binaural amplification. This requires that each ear receive sound from a different microphone *and* that those microphones be separated in space. There are many proponents of the use of binaural amplification with young hearing-impaired children, but objective data demonstrating its superiority over single channel amplification are hard to find. It has been my experience that while the use of two hearing aids, rather than one, may accelerate auditory development, it does not make the difference between success and failure. There are, however, only a few situations in which one would argue that it is better to fit one hearing aid than two.

developing the auditory perception of speech

In some respects, the sounds of speech are no different from the other environmental sounds to which the child is exposed. As you follow the suggestions in the preceding sections, there will, therefore, be many occasions on which speech is the natural source of sound for an auditory activity.

Obviously, however, the children stand to gain infinitely more from auditory speech perception than they do from the auditory perception of other sounds. You should therefore give top priority to the use of speech for auditory development. In addition, you should structure children's experiences of speech so that they can learn to appreciate its social and communicative significance. The following suggestions relate particularly to this last point:

Precede, and accompany with speech, all your interactions with the children. From this they should learn that the sounds of speech come from people and therefore signal the presence of a human being. Note that television and radio are counterproductive in this respect.

Ensure that all people who interact with the children do so to the accompaniment of speech. This will help them to associate particular voices with particular people.

Use, and encourage the use of, expressive speech. Let the tone of voice convey pleasure, happiness, disappointment, sadness, fear, anger, and so on. From this the child should learn to associate particular intonation patterns with particular emotional states.

Avoid the habit of keeping up an incessant monologue. Use speech instead to help establish a dialogue. Do not talk at the child but with him. Use short, simple sentences. Ask questions. Give instructions. Make comments. Accept the child's gestures and vocalizations as his or her contribution to the dialogue. Translate them into language and then respond. Take turns as the initiator and respondent. When the child tries to introduce a topic by pointing or gesturing, take that as a point of departure. In this way the child will learn

that speech is not just produced by people, but is used by them during communicative interaction;
that people's contributions to these interactions are broken down into short *sentence units;*
that sentence units have characteristic durational, rhythmical, and intonational properties;
that the function of a sentence unit (question, answer, command, comment, and so on) influences its intonational properties.

These are prelanguage lessons whose importance cannot be overstressed. Mothers instinctively interact with their babies in the ways just described. A hearing-impaired child who is two or three years old in other respects may still be a "baby" auditorily and linguistically and needs to be treated accordingly.

Give the child every possible opportunity to experience speech *by hearing alone.* You must remember that most of the features by which phrases, words, sounds, and intonation patterns are recognized can only be perceived auditorily. Therefore, the process of dissociation, which we discussed earlier as an aid to developing attention, becomes mandatory in the development of auditory speech perception. At a later stage, the addition of lipreading to the auditory sensations will provide both supplementary and complementary information and will play a key role in *language development*. In the early stages, however, lipreading does not contribute at all to *auditory development* and may even detract if it dominates attentional behavior.

The foregoing comment might prompt you to ask how we can develop speech recognition skills if we do not encourage auditory—visual association. The answer lies in the nature of words. Words do not have any intrinsic meaning and are not recognized for their own sake. They are labels for perceptual and conceptual categories. When we recognize a word, therefore, we are not doing so in terms of a set of speech movements. Our answer to the question, "What made the sound?" is an object, or an activity, or a category in our world model. By all means, therefore, we must allow the child to associate the sounds of words and phrases with the things they represent, but I repeat that we will not facilitate *auditory* development by associating the sounds of words and phrases with their visible movements.

developing the auditory control of speech

I deal with speech development in a subsequent chapter. This is an appropriate point, however, at which to deal with the establishment of a fundamental speech readiness skill.

An absolute essential for natural speech development is auditory-motor association. Just like their normally hearing counterparts, hearing-impaired children must learn the connection between the movements of their speech mechanisms and the sounds thus produced. The imitation of speech sounds is *impossible* without this basic skill.

You will recall that auditory-motor association is normally established during the first year of life through reflexive vocalization, purposeful vocalization, and exploration. (See Chapter Three.) The hearing-impaired child must be provided with the same opportunities for vocal play and babbling after he or she has been fitted with hearing aids. Anything you can do to encourage vocalization will help in this process—babbling games, singing, shouting, the *go game* with the child as instructor, and so on. If necessary, you can use sound level meters and visual voice indicators to initiate vocalization (See Figure 8–3.) Note that you will increase the likelihood of spontaneous or imitative vocalization if you simultaneously engage the child in a more general motor activity. For example, when coloring, say, "Round and round and round." When climbing the stairs, say, "Up, up, up." When pouring, say, "*Down* goes the water," and so on.

One of the difficulties in trying to establish auditory-motor association in a two or three year old is that of getting the child to attend to the sounds of his or her own speech. I have recommended the use of dissociation to encourage attending behaviors, but how can you dissociate the sound from the movement when the child is producing it? A possible solution is the use

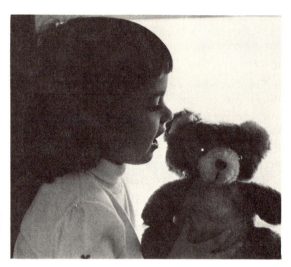

FIGURE 8–3 The Teddy Bear whose eyes light in response to sound provides one form of encouragement for vocalization and facilitates speech "readiness" by developing auditory-motor association.

of a tape recorder or a tape repeating device. Do not use these instruments, however, unless the child has the cognitive skills to understand what they do.

○ WHAT TO EXPECT

Hearing-impaired children differ widely in terms of auditory capacity. It therefore follows that given the same learning opportunity, different children will attain different levels of auditory performance. One way of looking at this is as a simple equation.

Auditory capacity X Learning opportunity = Auditory performance

If either quantity on the left of this equation is zero, the quantity on the right will be zero. Thus poor auditory performance can result from either poor auditory capacity or inadequate learning opportunity.

Failure to acknowledge this simple fact can lead to a variety of errors. On the one hand, a child with excellent auditory capacity may underachieve because of poor learning opportunities. On the other hand, the expectation of high auditory performance will result in frustration and disappointment for child, parents, and teachers if the basic auditory capacity is missing.

As a teacher, your responsibility is to aim for the establishment of an ideal learning opportunity, but not to make auditory performance the keystone of management. In other words, make auditory development one of your goals, but do not put all of your habilitative "eggs" in the auditory "basket."

predicting auditory performance

The foregoing comments prompt the obvious question, "Can we measure auditory capacity so as to predict auditory performance?" The answer, like so many in this field is a frustrating one—"Yes and no." The only measure of auditory capacity presently available to us is that of sensitivity—that is, the pure tone audiogram. It is, unfortunately, an incomplete measure. Thus, although we can make general predictions about the probability of certain auditory goals being accomplished, we cannot make absolute predictions of auditory performance for individual children.

Let me deal first with these general predictions.

mild or moderate losses

If the child's hearing loss is 60 dB or less, he or she will develop auditory skills without your intervention. There will, however, be deficits in certain areas, especially those related to attention and to the accuracy of speech perception and production. With good auditory management, you should expect to eliminate many of these deficits.

severe losses

Children with hearing loss between 60 dB and 90 dB, and no neural impairment, stand to gain most from good auditory management. Conversely, they stand to lose most from poor auditory management. You should expect such children to meet all of the goals listed at the beginning of this chapter, their performance being quantitatively only a little below that of children with normal hearing. Children with severe hearing losses should learn to localize and recognize sounds; they should learn to understand speech by hearing alone (for example, over the telephone) though not without difficulty; and their own speech should have normal rhythm and intonation with almost normal articulation. Such defects as occur in their speech should be limited to place of articulation errors, omission of weak consonants, and certain abnormalities of voice quality such as hypernasality and elevated pharyngeal resonance. *Without auditory learning opportunities, these children will function as if totally deaf.*

profound losses

Profound hearing losses cover the range from 90 dB to 115 dB or 120 dB. It is among children with profound losses that you will find the greatest variations of auditory capacity. It is also within this group that the pure tone threshold is least satisfactory as a predictor of performance. At one extreme, performance may be as good as that of children with severe hearing losses. In fact, with truly excellent auditory management, the boundary between severe and profound hearing loss should probably be shifted from 90 dB to 100 dB or even 105 dB. At the other extreme are children who have auditory sensitivity but cannot take advantage of it. This may be due to such things as tolerance problems, auditory adaptation, tinnitus, or poor discrimination of time and frequency differences. The performance of these children is indistinguishable from that of children with total hearing losses.

Between these two extremes are many children for whom the sense of hearing offers significant, though limited, benefits. Some may perceive (and, therefore, learn to produce) the rhythm and intonation of speech through hearing. Others may also learn to recognize vowels, and by integrating vision and hearing may learn to differentiate consonants on the basis of manner and voicing distinctions. Every effort should be made to capitalize on this capacity, although its limitations must be recognized.

total losses

The child with a total hearing loss does not experience auditory sensation, the only access to sound being through the sense of touch. Do not underestimate the potential value of this modality. It conveys time and intensity information and can, therefore, help the child recognize sounds with characteristic time patterns (for example, telephone bell, footsteps, and so on). Control of voicing can be acquired through the sense of touch, and tactile information about speech can supplement lipreading to the point where speech perception improves by 10 or 15 percent. But these are the limits. Totally deaf children cannot "hear" with their skin because it does not provide frequency information. They cannot recognize or reproduce the intonational and phonemic patterns of speech from purely tactile information. For these children, habilitation must proceed without the benefits of audition.

avoid negative predictions

If you wish to predict on the basis of threshold measurements, you should do so only in a positive sense—to confirm your commitment to auditory development. If, for example, a child's hearing loss is only 90 dB and there are no signs of neural involvement, you should feel confident in pursuing a program with a strong auditory emphasis.

You should, however, avoid negative predictions. Do not, for example, give up on hearing simply because audiometric results show the loss to be 115 dB. Remember, first of all, that hearing loss is not a perfect predictor. Remember also that behavioral measures of hearing loss often improve as the child's auditory development progresses. It is not uncommon for pure tone thresholds to improve by 10 dB or 15 dB once the child develops good listening skills. Do not assume absence of auditory capacity until all your best efforts have failed to produce auditory performance.

I am frequently asked, "How long should one keep trying before assuming that auditory capacity does not exist?" There is no simple answer to this, but I would estimate the proper time to be between one and two years. In the meantime, of course, you must ensure that the child's unfolding communicative needs are being met in nonauditory ways.

diagnostic teaching

It should be clear by now that the only sure way to determine auditory capacity is retrospectively. If, after exposure to ideal learning opportunity, the child's auditory performance is zero, we must assume that his or her auditory capacity is zero.

What I am advocating, therefore, is a process of diganostic teaching. Rather than prejudging what a child will or will not do, you should have a clear hierarchical model within which to evaluate the child's status and plan challenging learning experiences. The child's responses and rate of progress should be used to provide an increasingly detailed picture of his or her strengths and weaknesses.

○ DELIVERY

Until children are two or three years of age, auditory intervention will be the responsibility of the parents, almost exclusively. From about two and a half years on, they may benefit from individual sessions with a teacher, and when they are ready for group activities at around three years of age, these can be structured to provide motivation for, and reward of, auditory skill development.

With the emergence of early intervention programs there developed two philosophies about the type of professional who should handle auditory aspects of management, including those aspects involving parent education. On the one hand, it was thought that persons with training in education of the deaf would best be able to consider the needs of the whole child and to handle auditory development in this broader context. On the other hand, it was felt by many audiologists that they were the only persons whose training qualified them to deal with hearing aids, acoustics, and auditory training. In fact, the basic training of teachers of the deaf and of audiologists is uniformly inadequate as preparation for this work. Regardless of initial training, persons undertaking auditory management of young hearing-impaired children must prepare themselves by course work, independent study, and supervised experience. Only thus can they become qualified to deal properly with auditory needs within the context of counselling and education of parents and cognitive, social, emotional, and linguistic development of children.

○ EVALUATION

There are few formal tests that provide measures of auditory performance—fewer still if we consider only those which can be used with preschool children. If, therefore, you wish to describe the status of an individual child, the best tool is careful observation. I suggest you work within the framework of the objectives listed at the beginning of this chapter. As you ask whether the child meets each one, you should expand affirmative answers with examples of the behaviors on which your conclusion is based. You should also describe things the child cannot do, so as to provide an indication of quantitative performance within each qualitative objective.

When you come to the two speech-related objectives, some expansion is called for. Under objective 6—Will Use Hearing for the Perception of Speech—for example, I suggest:

will attend to the sounds of speech

will recognize speech as originating from people

will recognize individuals from the sounds of their voices

will respond to the emotional content of speech

will babble with the intonation contours of sentences

will attend to differences among words and phrases

will recognize words and phrases.

To provide quantitative information on this last objective, you may list the words recognized or report a percentage score on a formal test.

Under general objective 7—Will Use Hearing to Control the Production of Speech—I suggest:

will vocalize when the hearing aid is put on

will vocalize in imitation

will imitate the intonation patterns of sentences

will imitate vowel quality

will imitate consonants.

Under the last two entries, you can list which vowels and consonants are imitated when the model is provided auditorily. (See also Chapter Ten.)

You will notice the similarity between "will babble with the intonation contours of sentences" and "will imitate the intonation patterns of sentences," both of which relate to the child's production of normal intonation contours. There are, in fact, many speech perception skills that can only be evaluated in terms of their influence on speech production.

The purpose of auditory management is to provide learning opportunities so that auditory capacity can become auditory performance. If it is successful, the hearing-impaired children will develop auditory attention and recognition skills, they will be alerted by sounds, they will use sound to aid in the perception of space, and they will use hearing for the perception and production of speech.

To reach these goals we draw the child's attention to sounds, dissociate auditory sensations from other sensations, and provide multiple opportunities for the association of auditory sensations with other sensations. In addition, we use sound meaningfully to alert the child and to facilitate his interactions with his physical and social environment. In all of this work, top priority is given to the use of speech sounds, and every opportunity is provided for the child to learn the connection between his or her own speech movements and the resulting sound patterns.

Even with the most ideal learning opportunity, there will be big differences of auditory performance among individual children. This is due to differences of auditory capacity. These differences can be predicted partially, but not completely, from a knowledge of pure tone threshold.

Auditory management must occur within the broader context of habilitative intervention and must be undertaken by persons specially trained for this work. A degree in either audiology or education of the deaf is no guarantee of this training.

There are few formal tests of auditory performance. As you evaluate a child's auditory status, you should ask whether specific objectives have been met, supporting your conclusions with careful observations of behavior.

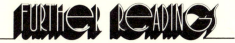

Erik Wedenberg has had considerable influence on the development of auditorily based programs. You should read his papers entitled "Auditory Training of Deaf and Hard of Hearing Children," (*Acta Otolaryngologica,* Supplement 94, 1951) and

"Auditory Training of Severely Hard of Hearing Pre-School Children," (*Acta Otolaryngologica,* Supplement 110, 1954). Other sources of information on the work of European pioneers are Henk C. Huizing's "Auditory Training," (*Acta Otolaryngologica,* Supplement 100, 1951), Edith Whetnall and Denis Fry's *The Deaf Child* (Chas. C Thomas, Springfield, Ill., 1971) and Alexander and Lady Ethel Ewing's *Hearing Impaired Children under Five* (Manchester University Press, Manchester, U.K., 1971).

Some of the better known American work is described by Ciwa Griffiths in *Conquering Childhood Deafness* (Exposition Press, New York, 1967) and by Doreen Pollack in *Educational Audiology for the Hearing Impaired Infant* (Chas. C Thomas, Springfield, Ill., 1970). I also recommend that you read Derek Sanders' *Aural Rehabilitation* (Prentice Hall, Inc., Englewood Cliffs, N.J., 1971) and Frederick N. Martin's chapter entitled "Speech Tests of Hearing—Age One through Five Years" in *Pediatric Audiology,* ed by F. N. Martin (Prentice-Hall, Inc., Englewood Cliffs, N.J., 1978). Patricia Elwood, Wayne Johnson, and Judith Mandell's *Parent-Centered Programs for Young Hearing Impaired Children* (Prince George's County Public Schools, Upper Marlboro, Md., 1977) is recommended, and Daniel Ling's chapter entitled "Auditory Coding and Recoding" in *Auditory Management of Hearing Impaired Children,* edited by M. Ross and T. G. Giolas (University Park Press, Baltimore, Md., 1979) is worth reading for its own merit as well as for the thorough review of the literature it contains.

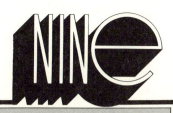

NINE

Cognitive and linguistic management

Language acquisition by the hearing-impaired child is one of the most important—and controversial—aspects of management. The importance of this topic lies in the central role played by language in determining the secondary consequences of hearing impairment. The controversy arises from the availability of several language systems—each with its own inherent strengths and weaknesses.

To say that cognition is a prerequisite for language development would be an understatement. Cognition is part of language. The symbols of language, like all symbols, have no meaning except in so far as they are used to stand for something else. In the case of language, the *something else* consists of the objects, events, attributes, rules, relationships, and concepts of an individual's world model. That is to say, the symbols of language stand for what a person *"knows"* about the world. (See Figure 9–1.)

It is true, of course, that once established, language can be used to enhance cognitive development, but in the infant and preschool child it is cognition that serves as the starting point for language. Without cognition there can be no language. Hence the inclusion of both topics in the present chapter.

○ EXPRESSION AND RECEPTION

Language competence reveals itself in two ways—through expression and through reception. *Expressive language behavior* involves the internal representation of thoughts by language patterns and the external representation of those language patterns by movement. *Receptive language behavior* involves the observation of the movements of another person and the interpretation of those movements in terms of the language patterns, and the thoughts, they represent.

competence

You should note that central to both types of behavior is a knowledge of the relationship between thoughts and language patterns. I refer to this knowledge as *language competence.* Expressive ability requires language competence plus certain specialized motor skills. Receptive ability requires language competence plus certain specialized perceptual skills. As you work

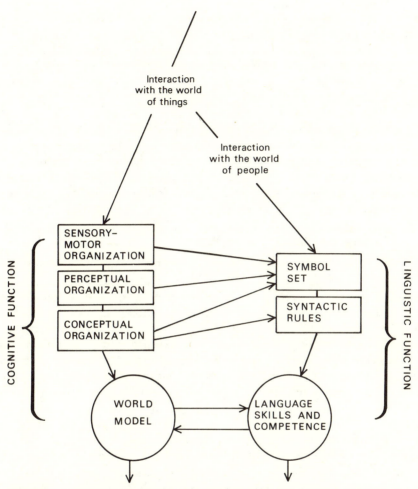

FIGURE 9–1 Illustrating the interdependence of cognitive and linguistic function in the developing child. This process is discussed at length in Chapter Three.

with the child you are, of course, concerned with development in all three areas. That is to say:

1. Learning the relationship between thoughts and language patterns.
2. Acquiring the motor skills for expression.
3. Acquiring the perceptual skills for reception.

focus of present chapter

I have discussed the acquisition of those skills necessary for perception of speech movements by means of hearing in Chapter Eight, and I deal with the acquisition of motor speech skills in Chapter Ten. The primary focus of the present chapter, therefore, is on establishing the connection between thoughts and language patterns. It should be obvious, however, that the hearing-impaired infant cannot acquire this important knowledge except through exposure to the language of others and through attempts to express his or her own thoughts by language. Once again, therefore, we are reminded of the impossibility of separating various aspects of development at the practical level.

I should also point out that hearing is only one of the possible modalities for perceiving speech which, in turn, is only one of the possible modalities for expressing language. In the present chapter I, therefore, discuss some alternatives to speech and hearing for language expression, reception, and acquisition. First, however, there are some additional aspects of expressive and receptive language behavior that need to be emphasized.

influence of situation on expression

When we receive a linguistically encoded message from another person, it is usually accompanied by many nonlinguistic sources of information. Examples are the temporal context, the situational context, previous messages, the common history of sender and receiver, tone of voice, gestures, facial expressions, and so on. When functioning expressively, we instictively take account of these nonlinguistic cues and tend to choose language patterns to convey information that is not available from other sources. The young child, for example, holding up a broken toy, will not say, "The toy is broken" since that is obvious for all to see. Rather he will say, "Annie broke it" (or simply "Annie") since this supplies the important missing information.

Similarly, we take account of the perceived cognitive and linguistic abilities of the recipient of our messages when choosing language patterns. The same thought may be expressed very differently to a baby, a toddler, a second grader, a teenager, an adult, a geriatric, a mentally retarded individual, a hearing-impaired child, or a foreigner. In the special case of babies and toddlers, we (again instinctively) break our rule of parsimony and deliberately parallel nonlinguistic information with language patterns since we want to help them learn our language—a point to which I shall return in a moment.

influence of situation on comprehension

I stated earlier that receptive language behavior involves interpreting the movements of another person in terms of both language patterns and thoughts. But which comes first—the language or the thought? To the extent that a person whose language competence is established can interpret the thought from nonlinguistic sources of information, he or she may do so and use the results to aid in the recognition of the language patterns. The capacity exists, however, to recognize the language independently of meaning, that is to perceive the language first and the thought second. Children who are developing language cannot do this. They must recognize the thought from nonlinguistic cues. If they happen simultaneously to be receiving equivalent language patterns, they then have the opportunity to associate thought and language. This is why we talk to babies about what we are doing, long before they have the necessary receptive language skills.

Eventually, children's world models become too complex and their communicative needs too great, for continued total reliance on nonlinguistic communication. It is at this point that they must begin to attend to the details of language patterns and to make and test inferences about the meaning of those patterns. This is where the real pressure for language development begins, and it is a situation we must exploit if we are to help the young hearing-impaired child develop language.

assessing competence

It should be obvious from the foregoing that the developing child, regardless of hearing status, encounters numerous situations in which the meaning of an utterance can be derived with little or no support from the language patterns themselves. In other words, the child's *message comprehension* ability may be very much better than his *language recognition* ability. We must therefore be very careful not to interpret a child's ability to understand everything we say as evidence of true language competence.

On the other side of the coin, it should also be obvious that a child's knowledge of the relationship between thoughts and language patterns may be inadequately reflected in expressive language ability—particularly in situations where proper motor control is prevented by such things as cerebral palsy or hearing impairment.

implications

To summarize the practical implications of the discussion so far,

1. The central ability that hearing-impaired children must acquire is that of representing thoughts, internally, by language patterns.

2. In addition, they must acquire specialized perceptual skills so as to have receptive language ability.

3. They must also acquire specialized motor skills so as to have expressive language ability.

4. Message comprehension can be accomplished first by nonlinguistic means, using language patterns in parallel to establish thought-language associations.

5. Language recognition can then be developed by using language patterns to convey increasing amounts of information that is not available from other sources.

6. Assessments of a child's true language competence may be unduly optimistic, if based solely on message comprehension, and unduly pessimistic, if based solely on expressive performance.

○ LANGUAGE MODALITIES

For children to acquire knowledge of language from the samples presented to them, it is necessary that the motoric code be fully *accessible*. That is to say, they must be able to detect all of the important movements and discriminate among movements carrying different information.

normal hearing

The criterion of *accessibility* is met for normal children by the speech code. Their sense of hearing permits them to detect and discriminate all of the important speech movements by virtue of the sounds those movements produce. Indeed, the characteristics of hearing have guided the evolution of speech codes (and perhaps even of the speech mechanism itself).

One of the consequences of hearing impairment is that the speech code is not fully accessible. Some speech movements may be undetectable to the hearing-impaired child and among those that are detectable, different movements may be indistinguishable.

methods

There are several ways of providing (or trying to provide) accessibility to the motoric codes of language for the child with imperfect hearing. Proponents of these various approaches fall into two general groups. In one group are people who insist on the exclusive use of the speech code, to which they offer direct access through residual hearing, vision, or touch, and indirect access through description or print. In the other group are people who favor the simultaneous use of manual symbols, either as a supplement to visible speech information or as a parallel, but independent, language system.

The "methods" used by the proponents of an exclusively oral approach include *the auditory-oral approach, the auditory approach, acoupedics* and so on. Those involving the use of manual supplements include *cued speech, the*

Rochester method, total communication and so on. I put "methods" in quotes since a method is by no means defined by its label.

Educators of the deaf have been bitterly divided on this issue for many years. While all agree that mastery of the speech code is desirable as a key to freedom of social and vocational choice in adult life, they do not agree on such things as the feasibility of such mastery for all hearing-impaired children; the social and emotional cost of pursuing this as an exclusive goal; and the interactions that take place when oral and manual codes are used together. I return to this topic at the end of the section. In the meantime, I need to discuss the various language codes and perceptual modes from the point of view of accessibility. My purpose is to provide a rationale on which choices may be made about the management of individual children.

auditory perception of speech

The important thing to remember about the auditory perception of speech is that accessibility depends on two things—the integrity of the hearing mechanism and the specific speech feature in question. Children with sensorineural hearing losses of less than 60 dB, for example, have almost full access to all speech features through hearing. When the loss is between 60 dB and 90 dB, all features except place of consonant articulation can be perceived auditorily. Most children with losses between 90 dB and 120 dB have access to rhythm and intonation through hearing, and many have access to vowel articulation and the manner and voicing of consonants. For the small percentage of hearing-impaired children who have no sense of hearing, auditory access to the speech code is, obviously, nil. Please note that when I discuss the use of residual hearing, I am always assuming the use of appropriate amplification and the prior development of auditory skills. (See Chapters Seven and Eight.)

visual perception of speech

The visual perception of speech—lipreading—is a very poor way of gaining access to the speech code. Most of the significant movements are invisible, and many of the visible movements are indistinguishable from one another. We cannot, for example, see movements of the breathing mechanism, the airstream, the vocal cords, or the velum. We can only see movements of the lips and jaw and at times, parts of the tongue. As a result, there is no access through vision to rhythm, intonation, voicing, or manner of articulation. Only place of articulation is accessible and that imperfectly.

The foregoing inventory seems, at first sight, incompatible with the fact that some people can "lipread." You should realize, however, that these are people who have already established language competence. With the help of situational, contextual, and other cues, they are able to attain high levels of *message comprehension* through lipreading in spite of their limited access to the motor patterns of spoken language. In contrast, the developing child needs full access to those patterns in order to *learn* the relationship between thought and language. The difference between the use of a perceptual modality for taking advantage of already established language competence and the use of the same modality for developing that language competence is extremely important and easily overlooked.

On a more positive note, I should add that many significant movements that are inaccessible by lipreading or residual hearing acting alone become accessible when the two are combined. Indeed, most children with severe hearing losses (less than 90 dB), and many with profound hearing losses (greater than 90 dB), can gain good access to the speech code through a combination of hearing and lipreading and can, therefore, be expected to acquire spoken language skills in a natural manner—by processing the meaningful speech input of others and experimenting with speech output.

tactile perception of speech

Tactile information about speech movements can be obtained in two ways: from the amplified acoustic output of a hearing aid and by manual exploration of the face and mouth of the talker.

The first technique offers extremely limited access and provides information on rhythm only. In conjunction with lipreading, however, tactile perception of the amplified acoustic speech signal may also provide access to manner of articulation and voicing of consonants. The acoustic stimulus may be detected by touch receptors in and around the ear if a standard, high powered, hearing aid is used. This is not, however, the most effective approach. The stimulus is more detectable and more discriminable if applied, through vibrational transducers, to more sensitive parts of the body, such as the fingers. Alternatively, the vibrations can be coupled to the skeleton at such places as the wrist, elbow, or collarbone and thus be distributed over a larger area. Please note that the tactile perception of amplified sound is in no way related to bone conduction hearing. In tactile perception, the vibrations are detected by touch receptors in the skin. In bone conduction hearing, the vibrations are detected by functioning hair cells in the cochlea. (See Chapter Two.)

It should be obvious that the approach just described would be used only with children who are without any useful hearing. You should also be aware that hearing aids with vibratory outputs and the means to couple them to hands or skeleton are not standardly available. They can, however, with a little ingenuity, be fashioned from existing components and materials. (See Appendix C.)

From time to time researchers and clinicians have aspired to teach deaf children to hear with their hands, using the techniques just described. This is an impossible goal. The sense of touch has extremely poor frequency discrimination and cannot, therefore, provide access to intonation and place of articulation. No amount of training can render the sense of touch even a close rival to hearing as a means of access to the speech code through acoustic signals. It should be used only as a supplement to lipreading and only for children with no residual hearing.

The second use of touch—for manual exploration of the speaker's face —offers considerable access to speech movements. By suitable hand placement one can feel the strength, location, and time characteristics of air flow; vibrations of the vocal chords during voicing; vibrations of the nose during nasalization of voiced sounds; and movements of the jaw. Manual exploration of the oral cavity provides some access to tongue position and configuration. The one important feature that cannot be perceived in this way is intonation.

There is, of course, a big drawback to the use of manual exploration. It is neither natural nor convenient for children to always have their hands on the faces of the people who are talking to them or on their own faces when talking to others. This technique does not, therefore, lend itself to application in the natural process of language acquisition. It can, however, be used very effectively in one-to-one teaching situations in which the focus is on the development of expressive skills as a stepping stone to language competence. More will be said about such *output-centered* approaches shortly.

Note also that for the child without either hearing or vision, manual exploration of the face is the only way of providing direct access to the speech code and must be used both for training and for one-to-one oral communication. In this context, the procedure is known as the *TADOMA* method.

description

I am using the word *description* to refer to all techniques that provide access to speech movements by telling children what they should do and how well they have done it. The information may be communicated verbally, by gesture, by models, or by diagrams. As with manual exploration, this technique would be reserved for one-to-one teaching situations in which the focus is on the development of speech output skills as a precursor to acquisition of language competence. Apart from its obvious clumsiness and slowness, the main drawback to the use of description is the fact that it is indirect. Children are not perceiving speech movements directly, either other people's or their own. Instead, they are being told about them and are, therefore, completely dependent on the reliability, consistency, and objectivity of another person.

print

Another indirect technique that can be used in the context of an output-centered approach is the early association between speech movements and print. By establishing a phoneme system and then teaching the child written symbols for phoneme categories, the teacher hopes to use expressive skills as a starting point from which to develop both language competence and receptive skills. Note, however, that the printed symbols are not being used to provide initial access to speech movement. They are used, instead, as an indirect form of access to movement patterns that have already been learned using residual hearing, and/or vision, and/or manual exploration, and/or description.

The early establishment of an association between print and speech movements carries some serious risks. These arise primarily from the fact that no system of orthography adequately encodes all of the significant speech movements. The most serious omission is of information about intonation and temporal patterns. The English system, for example, represents phoneme categories in a linear sequence, with spaces between words and the occasional capital, period, and comma to show syntactic boundaries. In real speech, the speech sounds flow into each other; there are usually no gaps between words; the durations of sounds and words change according to context and function; and syntactic boundaries are encoded by either gaps, durational changes, pitch changes, or a combination of the three. I believe that the early establishment of print as a means of indirect access to spoken language patterns has been a primary cause of the monotonous, choppy, arhythmic speech so widely reported in studies of deaf children. Thus, although print may aid in the acquisition of language competence, its premature use can jeopardize the eventual mastery of expressive speech skills.

a comment on output-centered approaches

At the beginning of this chapter I described the natural process of language development in which the child acquires language by progressing from message comprehension, to language competence, to mastery of receptive and expressive skills. I have now, however, introduced the concept of an output-centered approach in which the child progresses from expressive skills to language competence and receptive skills.

If you are working with hearing-impaired children whose sense of hearing, supplemented by vision, provides full access to the movements of the speech code, you may expect them to follow the natural pattern with no special emphasis on the "teaching" of expressive skills. Such children would normally have hearing losses that are less than 90 dB. With increasing degrees of hearing loss, it becomes increasingly necessary to use techniques that focus on the mastery of expressive speech skills. When the hearing loss is very profound, or total, the natural developmental process will lead to only crude levels of language competence, and it becomes mandatory either to use an output-centered approach or to introduce manual supplements.

manual cues

Oral educators of the deaf have, for years, used informal manual cues to remind children of previously learned motor skills and to resolve ambiguities in the speech code. Examples might be pointing to the larynx to indicate voicing; pointing to the nose to indicate nasalization; pointing to the nose with a shake of the head to indicate denasalization; and moving the hand horizontally to indicate duration. Such cues have never been standardized, however, and their use is sometimes discouraged on the grounds that they reduce the children's need to improve their receptive skills.

Using the rationale that full access to the speech code is necessary for language development, and unattainable by lipreading, educators in various countries have developed formal systems of manual cues. The systems have differed not only in terms of the choice of cues but also in terms of the information to be cued—the latter depending on the phonetic system of the language in question. Development of a system of cues for the English language was undertaken by Dr. Orin Cornett of Gallaudet College in the 1960s. His system is known as *cued speech.*

Cornett's system is strictly phonemic. That is to say, it provides cues to disambiguate those phoneme groups (for example, /p/, /b/ and /m/) that are indistinguishable from visual observation of speech movements. There is no attempt in cued speech to provide information about rhythm and intonation. (You will recall, however, that most hearing-impaired children can perceive rhythm and intonation auditorily.) You should further note that the cues are a supplement to lipreading. They provide information that cannot be seen by lipreading, just as lipreading provides information that cannot be obtained from the cues. Thus, for full accessibility to the phonemic code, the child must observe the speech movements *and* the cues. In this respect cues are different from fingerspelling and signing, in which accessibility to the language can be obtained from speech movements *or* manual symbols.

There is, of course, nothing in the manual cues to tell children about the speech movements they cannot see, unless these movements have already been taught and the association established. You cannot, therefore, expect the use of cued speech automatically to produce expressive speech skills in totally deaf children. They will spontaneously reproduce what they see—that is, the manual cues and the visible lip and jaw movements. Control of the invisible movements must be dealt with in specific, output-centered speech instruction.

The major advantage of cued speech for the child with little or no hearing is that it accelerates the acquisition of language competence by capitalizing on the natural development process. Children can learn language from all communicative interactions with their family and need not be left in the dark for a major portion of their day. For this advantage to be gained, however, it is obvious that the family must learn and practice the cueing system to the point where it becomes automatic and fluent. This in turn calls for a high degree of motivation on the part of all family members.

fingerspelling

Fingerspelling is a manual reencoding of print which itself is a reencoding of speech. It is more convenient than print as a medium for dialogue, though it cannot match the speed and efficiency of speech. The simultaneous use of speech and fingerspelling is known in the United States as *the Rochester Method,* and in the Soviet Union as *neo-oralism.*

Observation of fingerspelling provides children with direct and full access to the motor patterns of fingerspelling. They should, therefore, be expected to acquire language competence and expressive fingerspelling skills in a natural manner. Observation of fingerspelling does not, however, provide direct access to the motor patterns of speech. It may, like print, provide indirect access, but only if the child is first taught the motor skills of speech in an output-centered approach. Even then, the teacher must contend with the fact that the symbols of fingerspelling (like those of print) are only quasi-phonemic. That is to say, there is not a one-to-one correspondence between symbols and phoneme categories.

You should also note that the developing child need not attend to visual speech patterns if he or she has access to phonemic coding by means of fingerspelling. There is, therefore, no *intrinsic* need to master the expressive and receptive skills of spoken language if fingerspelling is used simultaneously. The need must be created extrinsically, by teachers and family. Thus the addition of fingerspelling to speech, while it may facilitate the acquisition of language competence and communicative skill *in the modality of fingerspelling,* by no means reduces the need for knowledge, expertise, and motivation from parents and teachers if competence and communicative skill *in the modality of spoken language* are also to be attained.

sign language

The manual symbols of sign language represent perceptual and conceptual categories within a world model. The signs of sign language are, therefore, analogous to the words of spoken language. Unlike fingerspelling, the process of signing involves no attempt to encode the movements of speech. You should note, however, that present day educators in the

United States are advocating, and using, sign languages that replicate the grammar and morphology of spoken language. The use of these signed English languages is beleived to be preferable to the use of American Sign Language, which has a grammar and morphology of its own. The hope is that mastery of spoken language, and/or its written derivative, will be acquired more easily if its form corresponds with that of the child's sign language. At the very least, there should be an avoidance of interference between spoken and signed languages with very different forms and structures.

By encoding at the concept level, sign languages achieve a speed and an efficiency similar to those of spoken language, and since the movements of sign language are fully accessible through vision, totally deaf children should have no difficulty acquiring competence and skills with signs—always assuming that they have lots of meaningful interaction with people who use sign language naturally and fluently with the children and among themselves. Early mastery of sign language should help to preserve developmental synchrony and promote ideal social, emotional, and communicative conditions for the development of spoken language skills. It is unreasonable, however, to expect spontaneous transfer from mastery of sign language to mastery of spoken language. If the child with a profound or total hearing loss is to develop competence and skills in spoken language, special output-centered techniques must be used. As with cued speech and fingerspelling, the demands on teachers and parents for skill, knowledge, and motivation are not diminished by the simultaneous use of signs and speech.

section summary

1. Mastery of a language code requires access to its movements.

2. Normal hearing provides full access to the movements of speech through the intermediary of the sounds they generate.

3. Defective hearing provides more or less access to the movements of speech, depending on the integrity of the hearing mechanism.

4. For any given hearing-impaired individual, auditory access to speech movements is different for different movements. In general, rhythm and intonation are most accessible while place of articulation of consonants is least accessible.

5. Vision provides very limited access to the movements of speech but full access to the movements of manual language codes.

6. Touch provides very limited access to the movements of speech by means of amplified sound but good access by means of manual exploration. Such exploration is best used for individual instruction in output-centered approaches.

7. Description is a poor form of indirect access by means of another person but again may be valuable in output-centered instruction.

8. Print can be used to provide access *after* the motor skills of speech have been learned in other ways. Its premature use with young children, however, carries serious risks for eventual speech mastery.

9. Cued speech provides a fully accessible movement code at a phonemic level, if the child watches both the cues and the speech.

10. Fingerspelling and sign language also provide fully accessible movement codes, and both can function entirely independently of speech.

11. The child with a hearing loss of less than 90 dB should have almost full access to the speech code through a combination of amplified hearing and lipreading and should, therefore, be able to acquire spoken language competence and skills in a natural manner.

12. The child with a hearing loss of more than 90 dB will generally require special instruction in the motor skills of speech if he or she is to master the speech code. This remains true whether or not manual supplements are used.

13. The addition of manual supplements should help the very deaf child to acquire language competence and communicative skills. These skills will help preserve developmental synchrony—especially of social and emotional function —and should, therefore, provide an excellent foundation for mastery of the speech code. Such mastery, however, will not occur spontaneously but will call for the same degree of skill, knowledge, and motivation from parents and teachers as if an exclusively oral approach were being used.

14. Whatever language modality is used with the child, it is imperative that the parents and family are, or become, fluent in it and comfortable with it.

○ METHODS DEBATE

In the previous section I have tried to discuss language modalities and methodologies in an objective manner. It is hard to preserve objectivity, however, if you are embroiled in the day-to-day lives of hearing-impaired children and their families, and even harder if you are the parent of a hearing-impaired child. In consequence, the issue of language modality is seldom argued at a rational level but is taken up in ideological and often vitriolic conflicts whose arguments are clouded by our concept of normalcy and our tolerance for deviation. Students, practitioners, and parents quickly find themselves under internal and external pressures to take sides in these disputes.

The most troublesome aspect of the methods dispute has been the unwritten, but implicit, assumption that there is a single method for all hearing-impaired children that can eliminate the secondary consequences of hearing impairment. This assumption is both unjustified and dangerous. To the extent that the child's hearing, with the assistance of vision, can provide almost full access to the speech code, the method of choice should be a natural, auditorily based, oral approach. If the child lacks that auditory capacity, there are two basic choices: Use an output-centered approach to speech instruction, and use expressive language as an inroad to language competence through the exclusive use of speech. Secondly, add manual supplements so that the child may develop one language modality naturally, and then treat mastery of the speech code as a separate process.

If you choose the former, you must be prepared to deal with the consequences of any undue delay in acquiring communicative skills; the child must have highly motivated and competent parents; and you must have considerable expertise in the areas of speech, hearing, and language. If you choose the latter, you may avoid some of the immediate consequences of language delay, but the child will still need highly motivated and competent parents—motivated enough to learn, and become fluent in, a new language —and you must still have considerable expertise in the areas of speech, hearing, and language.

In short, the acquisition of language by children with impaired or absent hearing presents serious problems to which there are no simple solutions. The very existence of a controversy over methods is a sign of our wish to deny this upalatable fact and of a need to find a focus for the anger we feel in response to the child and his or her deafness. If you are to be fully effective as a teacher and a counsellor, it is imperative that you explore and come to terms with your own feelings on these difficult issues.

For the remainder of this chapter I assume that speech is being used with and by the child, but I make no assumptions about the use or nonuse of manual supplements.

○ OBJECTIVES

If the cognitive-linguistic aspects of management are successful, the child will

1. Have a detailed and accurate world model that is appropriate to his chronological age and intellectual capacity.
2. Engage in dialogue with adults.
3. Understand and use words as symbols for various aspects of his or her world model.
4. Understand the meanings of sentences.
5. Modify and combine words so as to make sentences that convey his or her own thoughts and wishes.
6. Use language for a variety of purposes appropriate to his or her levels of cognitive and social development.

In short, the child will have things to talk about, people to talk with, a vocabulary, a grammar, and the ability to make them all work together.

general principles

As you work with children and their families, keep in mind the following principles, many of which I have already discussed:

1. *Before they can learn language patterns, children must know about the meanings those patterns will represent.* They will learn about meanings from exploration of, and interaction with, the world of things and the world of people.

2. *The proper forum for language development is dialogue.* This is an activity in which two people interact by passing messages back and forth. True dialogue requires that the participants take turns, not only as senders and receivers of messages, but also as initiators of new topics. Dialogue may occur both in play and in daily living activities.

3. *Before you can hope to introduce language as a mediator of dialogue, you must be able to engage the child nonlinguistically.* That is to say, you must have the personality, and be able to establish the rapport, that permit mutually satisfying, nonverbal play.

4. *Language patterns may first be introduced in parallel with nonlinguistic sources of information.* In this way, children receive the language from you and the meaning from the situation. They thus have the opportunity to learn the relationship between thought and language by association. It is imperative, however, that the children have full access to the movements of whatever language code you are using.

5. *You may then exert pressure to attend to language patterns by creating situations in which the nonlinquistic information carries only part of the message.* This requires the child to start making and testing hypotheses about the nature of the language code.

6. *When children express their thoughts nonlinguistically—by pointing, for example—accept the message, but reflect back the appropriate language pattern.* If they use imperfect language patterns, reflect back corrected ones. These activities allow for association between thoughts and language patterns, but now the thoughts are the child's own.

7. *As the children begin to acquire mastery of expressive language, you can exert pressure for its more frequent and accurate use by "failing" to understand messages from nonlinguistic cues alone.* In this way they are forced to attend to the details of their own utterances.

8. *During all of this work the primary purpose, as seen from the child's point of view, must be communication within the context of play (or daily living activities).* At no point should you convey to the child the idea that the primary purpose is language acquisition. You should not, for example, persist in activities that frustrate the children by virtue of their not understanding or making themselves understood. They must be allowed to succeed communicatively and to discover that greater successes occur with the use of language than without.

9. *For those children who lack the auditory capacity needed for full access to the speech code, you will need to introduce output-centered speech work, in parallel with the foregoing.* This work will involve imitation games and vocal play during which children can acquire control of their speech mechanism and learn the phonetic building blocks of the speech code. (See Chapter Ten.) This need exists regardless of method—oral, cued speech, Rochester Method, or Total Communication.

10. *Even if the child has the auditory capacity needed for full access to the speech code, this capacity must be developed through auditorily based speech and language activities.* (See Chapter Eight.) It may also be advisable to include some output-centered speech work, especially in the areas of consonant articulation.

developing a world model

During their waking hours, children receive sensory impressions from the materials, objects, events, and people in their environment. As they develop motorically, they also influence those materials, objects, events, and people by their own movements. The results of their activity provide them with more sensory impressions. In this way, children assimilate the raw material from which to construct their internal world models.

How do we ensure that the process just described take place as rapidly and as efficiently as possible? The first requirement is one of exposure. The children must have a stimulating environment—one that brings them into contact with a wide range of materials (water, sand, soap, cereal, string, paper, grass, concrete, and so on); a wide range of objects (cooking utensils, spoons, bowls, shoes, plants, trees, pets, bags, clothing, towels, cars, buses, and of course, toys); a wide range of events (cooking, eating, washing, dressing, shopping, visiting, walking, running, jumping, pounding, building, knocking down, throwing, catching, pushing, rolling, sleeping, laughing, crying, scolding, and so on); and a wide range of people (nuclear family members, relatives, friends, strangers, public servants, shopkeepers, and so on).

The second requirement is one of exploration. The children must be able to interact with their environment and to find out what happens (both physically and socially) when they hit, push, pull, walk over or into, bite, suck, "talk" to, or otherwise attempt to influence the materials, objects, and people they encounter.

The third requirement is for an expanding environment. Although children need a base in the reliable, the familiar, and the predictable, they must also be challenged constantly by new things, new experiences, new activities, and new people. It is the challenge of the unfamiliar that provides the stimulus for cognitive growth.

But exposure, exploration, and novelty are not enough. For optimal value, the child's experiences must provide problems to be solved. In fact the child, given a sufficient range of options, will usually select the most challenging activities—emptying the wastepaper basket, unwinding a ball of wool, sitting on the cat, and so on. In this connection it is well to give special consideration to the choice of toys and play materials. It is almost a cliché that the child's parents are upset by his or her preference for a spoon and a couple of lids over the bright, attractive, but inherently boring, toy on which they have lavished much time and expense. The most suitable toys are those that provide

> multiple possibilities for play
>
> freedom for the child to be creative
>
> opportunities for motoric involvement
>
> the need for attention to similarities and differences of shape, size, and color
>
> problems to be solved.

As children grow older, they should also have toys that can be used as symbols for the objects and people of their environment—toy animals, people, cars, houses, and so on, as well as general purpose building blocks. These give children opportunities for reenactment, rehearsal, and fantasy, as well as preparing the way for the use of the more esoteric symbols of language.

In selecting toys, or advising parents on their selection, you must remember that toy manufacturers are subject to the pressures of the marketplace and that their consumers are adults, not children. Look for the products of companies that have taken their role seriously enough to make toys that are both appealing to the adults who must buy them and appropriate to the children who will receive them. Note also that children's needs change with age and that several manufacturers provide an indication of the age range for which their various products are suitable.

In summary, the child's waking hours should be filled with rich and stimulating experiences that provide a balance between the familiar and the novel and allow for exploration, problem solving, abstraction, and symbolism. In this kind of environment, the child should develop an accurate and detailed model of the world and, therefore, have a lot to talk about. Your greatest asset for this phase of your work will be the ability to see the world from the child's perspective. Your greatest successes will come when you have helped parents do the same.

establishing dialogue

Children acquire language during interactions with people who already use language. Our concern in this chapter is with the form of those interactions—specifically with tailoring them so that language acquisition can occur as effectively and as efficiently as possible.

Your first, and most basic, responsibility in relation to language development is to establish *dialogue* between yourself and the child, and more importantly between parents and child. Please note that I am using the term *dialogue* in a very general sense, without reference to the use, or nonuse, of language as a medium for communication. Perhaps the concept of *dialogue without language* seems like a contradiction in terms, but all of the characteristics of dialogue can be established without language. In fact, I believe they *must* be established if the nonverbal or preverbal child is to acquire language.

There are basically two contexts for dialogue with a very young child: activities of daily living (that is, necessary interaction), and shared play (that is, optional interaction). It is, of course, questionable whether such a dichotomy exists for the child, but it certainly exists for parents, many of whom need to understand that they can influence language development in both contexts. Note that there is a third context for dialogue: Conversation —that is, interaction mediated entirely by language. This last corresponds more closely to the usual concept of dialogue, but it does not become an option for the child until he or she has attained considerable mastery of language.

What are the characteristics of dialogue?

1. It involves two people.
2. Each person has a need, and/or a desire, to interact with the other.
3. At any given moment there is a *topic* that occupies the thoughts of both people.
4. Messages about the topic are passed back and forth, one person acting as *talker* while the other acts as *listener.*
5. The partners take turns at being talker and listener.
6. The partners take turns at initiating new topics.

In conversational dialogue, the messages are encoded in language. In dialogue without language, the messages may be conveyed by vocal or manual gestures, pointing, shaking or nodding the head, changes of facial expression, drawing attention to similarities and differences, pantomime, and so on. Often the nature of the message is obvious from context or from previously shared experiences, in which case the "talker" need only indicate that a message is being sent. With small babies, there may be no messages as such—except perhaps, "I want to keep this dialogue going."

In listing the characteristics of dialogue, I have raised several points that are worthy of elaboration. Note, for example, the fact that two people are involved. A child cannot establish dialogue with a television set. Note also the reference to a *need* and *desire* for interaction. The dialogue must be inherently meaningful to the child, as well as to the adult. There must also be a sense of empathy, trust, mutual interest, and mutual enjoyment. If you wish to establish dialogue with children, you must be able to make them feel secure, they must know that you care about them and their perspective, and you must be fun to be with. You cannot of course *fake* it. You must *be* trustworthy, you must *be* interested in the child as a person, rather than as a problem, and you must enjoy interacting with children. A teacher who cannot get along with children is about as effective as a pen without ink. (I should acknowledge, however, that children's personalities differ as much as do those of adults. Establishment of rapport often depends on matching of personalities, rather than on the separate characteristics of each one.)

The last issue of importance in describing dialogue is that of *turn taking,* —not only as senders of messages, but also as initiators of new topics. Turn taking implies shared control, and it is on the issue of control that most problems between teacher and child, or parent and child, hinge. If dialogue is to take place, children must be allowed to share in its direction—they must be active participants with a sense of equality of responsibility. Children who are denied their proper role can react in three ways:

1. Withdraw and refuse to interact.
2. Become purely passive participants.
3. Attempt to seize complete control.

Any of these reactions destroys the essence of the dialogue and seriously diminishes the opportunities for language acquisition. These reactions may be precipitated by teachers who are excessively directive and who take no account of the child's perspective. They may also be precipitated by parents in reaction to the guilt, fear, anger, and impotence they experience in relation to the child and his or her deafness. At one extreme are those parents who are afraid to direct or discipline. At the other are those parents who take on the cause of speech and language development to the complete exclusion of the child as an individual.

How do you set about establishing dialogue with a young child and helping the parents do the same? This question reminds me of a story concerning a well-known jazz musician who, when asked by an admirer to define rhythm, replied, "Lady, if ya gotta ask, ya ain't got it!" Most parents, indeed most people, know instinctively how to interact with young children. If, because of their cultural backgrounds or some lack of social and emotional integrity, they are unable to do so, there is little to be accomplished by way of instruction. The best you can hope for in parent guidance is to help remove or prevent those barriers to spontaneous interaction that arise from the mourning process and the failure of the child to respond to the parents' input at the appropriate age. Parents need to be reassured that they are competent to manage a hearing-impaired child, that the best thing they can do is to relax and enjoy their child, and that they need not feel embarrassed about playing and talking in ways that are appropriate to the child's language age rather than to his or her chronological age.

Similarly, if you yourself are having difficulty establishing dialogue, you should ask whether you are allowing your concern over language development to stand in the way of your prior need to relate to children as children. Until you can play with them and find mutual satisfaction in doing so, you do not have the proper conditions for language intervention.

developing vocabulary

As young children develop, they first organize their experiences into a world model of people, objects, and events. They later reorganize this world model into one of space, time, attributes, rules, and relationships. The first might be called a *perceptual world model*—the second, a *conceptual world model.*

During dialogue a child has a need both to inform other people about what is uppermost in his or her consciousness and to determine what is uppermost in theirs. This is the point at which *words* are needed to serve as symbols for various aspects of perceptual and conceptual world models. Your responsibility is to teach the particular words that are in current use in the immediate social environment.

As you interact with the children during play, or daily living activities, let them hear and see the words that are appropriate to the messages you are conveying. In this way they will have an opportunity to associate words with what those words stand for. When you introduce vocabulary, keep in mind the following principles:

1. The words should refer to things that are relevant to the child's everyday needs and experiences, that is, they must be potentially useful to him or her.

2. It should, at first, be obvious to the child what a new word stands for.

3. While there is no harm in the child receiving the words in isolation, he or she must also experience them in various sentence contexts. This is because the duration, intonation, and even the articulation of a word can change dramatically with its position and function in a sentence.

4. Give the child many opportunities to experience each word. You can, to a certain extent, make up for restricted accessibility by increased exposure.

5. Avoid the use of pronouns until the child has the word in his or her vocabulary.

6. Ensure that the child has access to the movement patterns that are essential to the production of the words.

The second step in vocabulary development is to use words to convey information that cannot be conveyed nonlinguistically. Suppose, for example, you are playing with the child, and you start to hunt around, look puzzled, and say, "I need the ball. Where is the ball?" There is lots of nonlinguistic information to suggest you are looking for something, but the child must use the language patterns to determine exactly what. If, after a couple of attempts, he or she cannot determine what you want, you should provide the information by a gesture, a picture, or by finding the ball yourself. Incidents like this oblige the child to pay attention to the details of language and exert a powerful, but subtle, pressure in the direction of language acquisition.

As you attempt to develop a receptive vocabulary in this way, keep in mind the following principles:

1. Withhold nonlanguage cues until the child has had an opportunity to process the language cues.

2. If he or she does not arrive at the correct interpretation quickly, avoid prolonging embarrassment or a sense of failure. Give the information nonlinguistically. By trying, the child will have learned something and increased the chances of success the next time. If you persist in offering messages he or she cannot comprehend, you will create anxiety and destroy confidence— both of which will be ultimately counterproductive.

3. You may begin by presenting the words in prominent positions in short sentences—even in isolation—but, as the child acquires more skill, you should give him or her the opportunity to recognize them in less prominent positions and in longer sentences.

The third step in this process relates to the child's own use of words. Even without a receptive or expressive vocabulary, the child will contribute his or her share to nonlinguistic dialogue. You will usually be able to determine from context and from gestures what message is being sent. Respond accordingly, but first speak for the child—using the key vocabulary word in a prominent position (for example, "*Open? Open* the box. There, I *open*ed the box. The box is *open.*" and so on). There is no need at this point for the child to use the word. What you are providing is another opportunity for association between word and meaning.

The fourth step involves applying pressure in the direction of expressive vocabulary development. Here you are treading on dangerous ground since you run the risk of teaching the child that words are simply things spoken by teachers (or parents) for repetition by children in order to gain social approval.

To the extent that the child has access to the movements of other people's speech, he or she should begin to experiment with the production of words spontaneously. If you have used an output-centered approach to mastery of speech skills, you will already have established imitation as an enjoyable and unthreatening activity. (See Chapter Ten.) In either case, you can encourage the child to produce words by momentarily delaying your responses to requests. (For example, if the box to which I just referred contains something of extreme interest to the child, a pregnant pause after "Open the box" should be a powerful motivator for imitation.) As in the case of language recognition, however, you must not frustrate the child by demanding imitation and making an issue out of it if the response is not immediate.

As the child begins to experiment with an expressive vocabulary, you can encourage development in two ways—increased accuracy and practical use. If his or her first attempts are only approximations, accept them, but repeat the words correctly. Once again, you can encourage imitation of the corrected patterns, but with care.

Once you know that certain words are in the child's expressive vocabulary, encourage their use by temporarily failing to understand nonlanguage cues. This a powerful way of applying pressure for language output since the focus is on its usefulness rather than on its form. The same general word of caution must be applied, however. Do not back yourself into a corner by demanding language use. Once you convey to the child the idea that your interactions exist only as a forum for language acquisition, you are in danger of destroying the trust that is fundamental to the establishment of dialogue.

developing sentence comprehension

Sentence comprehension is considerably more difficult than word recognition for several reasons:

1. It requires recognition, and short term storage, of several words.

2. The thought represented by a sentence involves not only the meanings of several words but also the relationships among them.

3. The clues to these relationships are contained partly in the words (especially the function words), partly in their sequence (that is, word order), and partly in modifications (pluralization, changes of verb tense, and so on). The rules for this aspect of encoding vary from language to language and are, to a considerable extent, arbitrary. That is to say, there is no good reason for doing things a given way in a given language—we just have to learn that way.

4. Sentence comprehension skills cannot be acquired by simple association, since most of the sentences we receive are new to us. The words may be familiar, but the particular selection and sequence is not. The meaning of a sentence must, therefore, be arrived at by a process of deduction, using our knowledge of word meanings, grammatical rules, and context. Our knowledge of the grammatical rules must be arrived at by a process of induction —abstracting general relationships from specific examples.

It is a testimony to the capacity of the human brain that normal children acquire full mastery of sentence comprehension, and production skills, by the time they are five, six, or seven years old (depending on the complexity of the language they must learn).

How do we help a young hearing-impaired child master the skills of sentence comprehension? First, we need to understand that the relationships conveyed by function words, word order, and word changes must exist already in the child's mind. In other words, by enhancing cognitive development and problem solving skills, we lay the groundwork for sentence comprehension, just as we did for vocabulary development.

Second, we need to structure our dialogue so that the information on relationships is conveyed less and less by context and more and more by language. For example, once the child is understanding messages from one key word plus nonlanguage cues (for example, holding out your hand and saying, "Give me the *car*"), you must plan your utterances so that comprehension requires recognition of two key words, three key words, and so on (for example, "*Give* me a *yellow crayon*" without holding out your hand). By judicious control of nonlanguage cues and message complexity, you can put pressure on the child to seek more information from the language patterns.

As with word recognition, you must exercise caution

1. Ensure that the child does in fact have access to the language patterns to which he or she must attend.

2. Give the child a chance to process the more complex language but provide the security of knowing that the nonlanguage cues will follow if the message is not understood. Do not create anxiety by unnecessary continuation of confusion.

Remember always that the *capacity* for language acquisition is unimpaired by damage to the hearing mechanism. Your responsibility is to overcome the problems of limited access by increasing both the amount of language input and the effectiveness of that input.

developing sentence production

As the child begins to evolve grammatical rules and to apply them in language output, accept the meanings but reflect back utterances that are more correct. For example:

> *Child:* Dolly cry!
>
> *Teacher or parent:* Yes, the dolly is crying.
>
> *Child:* Mommy home car?
>
> *Teacher or parent:* Will Mommy take you home in the car?
> No! You'll go home on the bus.

To the extent that the child will repeat the corrected language pattern without signs of frustration and without undue interruption of the dialogue, this should be encouraged. Again, however, you should avoid causing anxiety or creating the impression that the form of language is more important than its function.

developing multiple uses of language

Expressive language serves many functions. For example,

> Controlling the behavior of others ("Stop that!")
>
> Providing missing information ("Jeremy hit me!")
>
> Reminiscing about shared experiences ("We saw a dog at Grandma's house.")
>
> Asking questions ("Why is the lady crying?")
>
> Answering questions ("Because I don't like him!")
>
> Expresing feelings ("I'm mad!")
>
> Commenting on the world model ("A nest is a bird's house.")
>
> Commenting on language ("Wriggle is a funny word.")

These functions are inherent, not in the nature of language, but in the nature of humankind. In their interactions, even nonverbal children will engage in all of these functions (with the possible exception of the last). You do not, therefore, need to teach the children to ask questions, control behavior, and so on, but you do need to help them discover that language can be used for all of these purposes. The basic techniques for this are to use language yourself for various purposes, and when the children communicate nonverbally, to repeat their messages for them in linguistic form. Let me remind you again that the thing to avoid is teaching the child that language is something uttered by teachers for repetition by children in order to gain social approval.

○ WHAT TO EXPECT

The neurologically intact child with a moderate or severe hearing loss (90 dB or less) should be expected to follow a developmental course that is close to normal—assuming, of course, that the auditory goals of the previous chapter have been met. Among children with profound hearing losses (90 dB to 120 dB), there will be some who will function in the same way, some who follow the normal course but with significant delays, and others who will function as if totally deaf. Degree of hearing loss is, of course, not the sole determining factor. Parental attitudes and abilities, age of detection, and personality and language aptitude of the child will also play critical roles.

The totally deaf, or nonauditory child, even though neurologically intact, cannot gain full access to the spoken language code. Cognitive development can proceed normally during the preschool years, and an extensive receptive vocabulary can be established by lipreading—permitting message comprehension in situational context. If, however, a purely natural approach is used, spoken vocabulary, sentence recognition, and sentence expression will fall far short of normal function by the time the child is four or five years of age. If the child is exposed to manual supplements, the problem of accessibility is largely resolved. Let me emphasize again, however, that while this may deal with problems of language development in a general sense, the specific problem of developing receptive and expressive skills in the spoken modality will remain and will still need to be addressed through an output-centered approach.

If you are dealing with a child whose receptive and expresive language skills are far below your expectations, try to determine the cause. Is he neurologically intact? Are his problems social and emotional in nature? Has he been turned off by early exposure to activities that focussed on the form of language without regard to its use? A knowledge of cause does not necessarily determine treatment, but it can often reveal the inadequacies of current approaches. If, for example, the child's problem is one of anxiety about verbal communication, it may be counterproductive to apply more pressure in the area of language until this problem is resolved. At the same time, an awareness of the factors operating in one child may help you to avoid creating similar problems in other children.

○ DEALING WITH LANGUAGE DELAY

What are the immediate consequences of delayed language development? It might be assumed from what I have written so far that the possession of language skills does not become important until the end of the preschool years. This is not so. The child who is *acquiring* language is also *using* it to deal with the physical and social environment. He or she is enlisting help, making feelings known, establishing relationships, preparing for the unfamiliar, and so on. The child who cannot use language to meet his or her unfolding needs must have nonverbal alternatives. Otherwise there will be frustration and unhappiness, resulting in withdrawal, rigidity, or tyranny.

The purpose of the foregoing paragraph is to emphasize your need, not only to facilitate language development, but also to address the consequences of language delay. Your goal should be to help the parents reduce the need for language to the point where the child's environment is challenging but not overwhelming. The key to this control is predictability. To the extent that the child's daily life follows an established routine, to the extent that people respond to him in consistent ways, to the extent that he knows that certain causes always produce certain effects, the child's need for language diminishes. You must realize (and help the parents realize) that language deals with information and information deals with the uncertain. If we reduce uncertainties in the environment, the child's basic needs can be met more fully, despite the inadequacies of his or her language. The result will be a happier, more self-confident child who is easier to live with, and more fun to be with. This does not contradict statements made at the beginning of the chapter about the need for change and variety. In fact, children need a balance between certainty and uncertainty so that they may use existing skills to meet current needs and develop new skills to meet future needs.

○ EVALUATION

Descriptive evaluations of progress in this area can be based on the objectives given earlier in the chapter. I suggest you rephrase them in the form of questions.

1. Does the child demonstrate age-appropriate cognitive skills? Supplement your answer with descriptions of his or her abilities and behaviors. Where possible, use standardized tests or rating scales. Take care, however. Most tests of cognition rely on the child's spoken language output to assess internal thinking processes. When dealing with hearing-impaired children, you must look for tests or test items that are not verbally based.

2. Does dialogue take place between you and the child and between parents and child?
    Is the control of messages shared?
    Is the control of topics shared?

3. Does the child recognize words as labels for
    Objects and people?
    Events?
    Attributes?
    Supplement your answer with a list of receptive vocabulary while this is still small (say 100 words or less). Use standardized tests (for example, the *Peabody Picture Vocabulary Test*) when appropriate. Specify whether the child recognizes the words by hearing alone; lipreading and hearing; hearing and cueing; fingerspelling; signing; and so on. Specify whether recognition requires the support of situational context.

4. Does the child express words as labels for
    Objects and people?
    Events?
    Attributes?

Again, supplement your answer with a list of expressive vocabulary while this is still small (say 100 words or less). Specify the modalities used for expression—speech; speech and cues; fingerspelling; signing, and so on. Comment on intelligibility (a) to persons familiar with the child, (b) to persons unfamiliar with the child.

5. Does the child understand sentences that require the recognition of
   One word?
   Two or more words?
   To answer this question, you must think carefully about situational context. If, for example, it is close to the time of day when the child would normally go outside, "Get your coat" requires only recognition of the last word. If it is "coat-getting" time and you routinely require children to bring each other's coats, "Get Mary's coat" requires only recognition of the middle word. If, on the other hand, children routinely get their own coats and one day you unexpectedly say to George, "Get Mary's coat," he must recognize and relate two words for message comprehension.

6. Does the child use sentences consisting of two or more words? Supplement your answer with examples.

7. Does the child use language to
   Control the behavior of others?
   Provide missing information?
   Ask questions?
   Answer questions?
   Make statements about his or her world model?
   Make statements about language?
   Give examples of the language used. If the child uses nonverbal means of meeting these needs, give examples of these too.

The foregoing is primarily a descriptive evaluation, designed to emphasize the global nature of cognitive-linguistic development and perhaps to reveal weaknesses in programming. You may also wish to perform more quantitative evaluations, using either norm-referenced or criterion-referenced tests.

Cognition provides the basis for language. Additional requirements are

1. Knowledge of the relationship between thought and language
2. Expressive skills
3. Receptive skills

Estimates of language competence may be unduly optimistic if based solely on message comprehension ability and unduly pessimistic if based solely on expressive ability.

Language acquisition requires access to the language movements of self and others. Normal hearing provides access to the movements of spoken language through the medium of sound. Methods of providing access to language for the hearing-impaired child fall into two types: those that seek access to spoken language exclusively, using residual hearing, vision, and touch, possibly supported by description and print; and those that supplement speech movements with visually accessible hand movements. The use of manual supplements can largely resolve the problems of acquiring language per se, but if mastery of language in its spoken modality is expected, skillful, output-centered teaching is required—especially for the profoundly deaf. This requirement exists regardless of the use or nonuse of manual supplements.

The objectives of cognitive-linguistic management are

1. An appropriate world model
2. Establishment of dialogue
3. Receptive and expressive vocabulary
4. Sentence comprehension
5. Sentence production
6. Appropriate language use

These goals are accomplished through experiential enrichment, play dialogue, the use of language in parallel with nonverbal messages, the introduction of activities that require attention to the details of language, and the reflective reinforcement of the child's language output.

The negative effects of language delay can be offset, partially, by predictability and routine. Care must be taken, however, not to remove the need for language altogether.

Evaluation can be formal or informal and should cover cognition, dialogue, vocabulary, sentence comprehension, sentence production, and language use.

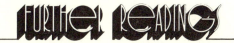

FURTHER READING

Richard and Laura Kretschmer's *Language Development and Intervention with the Hearing Impaired Child* (University Park Press, Baltimore, Md., 1978) is a challenging but valuable text and an excellent source of references. Dennis Fry's chapter on "The Role and Primacy of the Auditory Channel in Speech and Language Development," in *Auditory Management of Hearing Impaired Children,* edited by M. Ross and T.G. Giolas (University Park Press, Baltimore, Md., 1978) is also recommended.

Much of the literature on language teaching focuses on school age children. Some specific references to early language training are K. B. Horton's, "Infant Intervention and Language Learning" in *Language Perspectives,* edited by R. Schiefelbusch and L. Lloyd (University Park Press, Baltimore, Md. 1974), W. N. Northcott's, *Curriculum Guide: Hearing Impaired Children (0–3 years) and their Parents* (A. G. Bell Association for the Deaf, Washington, D.C., 1977), and A. Simmons-Martin's, "Early Management Procedures for the Hearing Impaired Child" in *Pediatric Audiology,* edited by F. N. Martin (Prentice-Hall, Inc., Englewood Cliffs, New Jersey, 1978).

For information on cued speech you should read Mary E. Henegar and R. Orin Cornett's, *Cued Speech—Handbook for Parents,* (Gallaudet College, Washington, D. C., 1971), and recommendations about play material can be found in Barbara Kaban's *Choosing Toys for Children* (Schocken Books, 1979). For a critical survey of standardized tests, I refer you to Richard Merson, Barbara Fishman, and Shirley Fowler's *Central Institute Test Evaluation Booklet* (Central Institute for the Deaf, St. Louis, Mo., 1976).

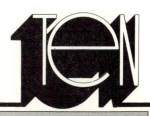

ten

Speech management

In this chapter I deal with the development of motor speech skills. Under normal circumstances, the sense of hearing plays a double role in speech acquisition. It is the *input* modality by which the speech patterns of others are perceived, and it is the *feedback* modality by which control of the child's own speech is established. Impairment of hearing implies the use of special techniques to ensure speech development.

○ GENERAL CONSIDERATIONS

aspirations

How reasonable is it to expect mastery of complicated motor skills when the primary input and feedback modality is absent or defective? You will not need to search very far to find educators who will answer, "Totally unreasonable" and others who will say, "Perfectly reasonable," each basing his or her opinion on professional experience.

Before offering my own opinion, I would like to clarify the concept of *mastery.* Ideally we would like hearing-impaired children to develop *normal speech patterns*—that is to say, patterns that fall within the range of those used by normally hearing talkers. A more realistic goal, especially for children with profound hearing losses, is the development of *effective speech patterns*— that is to say, patterns that permit listeners to recreate the intended linguistic structures. There are, of course, different degrees of effectiveness. At the highest level, the child's speech would be intelligible to strangers without the support of context. At the lowest level, the child's speech would require contextual support, and even then would be intelligible only to family and teachers.

It has been my experience that all children whose hearing losses are no greater than 90 dB can acquire normal, or near normal, speech patterns. Most of the children whose hearing losses exceed 90 dB can learn highly effective speech patterns which are intelligible to strangers. Within this second group at least 50 percent can acquire normal patterns of rhythm and intonation, despite abnormalities of vowel and consonant articulation. There are, however, certain prerequisities:

1. Absence of neurological impairments.
2. Early intervention.

3. Proper amplification.
4. Effective auditory development.
5. Parents who are informed, supportive, and involved.
6. Skillful teaching.

input-centered vs. output-centered approaches

Some educators prefer an *input-centered approach* to early speech development. That is to say, they expose the children to as much speech as possible, in the expectation that they will follow a normal developmental course—assimilating input for several months and then experimenting with output. Other educators argue against this on the grounds that it does nothing to resolve the problems of developmental asynchrony, discussed in Chapters One and Three. Their solution is to use an *output-centered approach* in which the child is engaged in activities specifically designed to elicit and consolidate correct speech habits as soon as possible.

In practice, the dichotomy is not as severe as the foregoing might suggest. Children who are slow to respond to an input-centered approach may well find themselves under pressure from their teachers to produce speech, and a good output-centered approach incorporates the development of receptive skills.

As you might expect, neither approach can be considered appropriate for all children. Those with moderate and severe hearing losses often respond well to an input-centered approach since, with proper audiological and auditory management, they can gain almost full access to the acoustic patterns of speech and can, therefore, follow a relatively normal developmental schedule. In contrast, children who must rely on vision for all or most of their speech input have poor access to the speech patterns of others and even poorer access to their own. For such children, an emphasis on output may well become mandatory. A word of warning, however. An output-centered approach can only be effective if the child is taken through carefully graded steps of steadily increasing difficulty, at a rate that permits mastery of skills at one level before moving on to the next, and in an environment that ensures relaxation, freedom from anxiety, and a maximum of positive reinforcement. Your skills, knowledge, and sensitivity will be tested in this area as in no other aspect of your teaching.

global vs. analytic approaches

Another source of disagreement among educators concerns the best starting point for speech work in terms of the size of linguistic structure. In a *global approach* children first learn to produce the rhythmic and melodic patterns of sentences, the expectation being that they will gradually refine their articulation as they become aware of the finer details of speech. In an *analytic approach,* children first master the basic sounds of speech, the expectation being that they will learn to build sounds into syllables, syllables into words, and words into sentences.

In general, the input-centered approaches tend to be global, whereas the output-centered approaches tend to be analytic. The danger, in both, is of inadequate follow through. Children taught *only* globally develop errors of articulation that resist later remediation, and children taught *only* analytically seldom learn to produce normal rhythm and intonation, even if they have the necessary auditory capacity. The implication is that early speech work must address both global and analytic needs. The two aspects of speech production must develop hand in hand.

You should note further that the global features of speech are more easily perceived auditorily than are the analytic features. The same child may, therefore, benefit from an input-centered approach when learning to produce sentence patterns, while requiring a more output-centered approach for mastery of vowel and consonant articulation.

cued speech

The use of manual cues to supplement speech input does not automatically help the child develop new speech output skills. There is nothing in the cues to tell the child how to produce speech sounds, nor do his own cues provide feedback to let him know whether he has produced the sounds correctly. On the positive side, however, you should note that once a system of vowels and consonants has been mastered, manual cues can be used to provide information about the phonemic structure of new words, and about phoneme omissions and substitutions in the child's own speech. Oral educators of the deaf have, in fact, used informal manual cues in this way for many years.

print

By reencoding speech in written form we can, in theory, provide hearing-impaired children with full access to the language system. As with cues, however, print does not help in the acquisition of the motor skills of speech. Its role in speech instruction is limited to providing input about the phonemic structure of new words and feedback about phoneme omissions and substitutions. It can only play this role *after* the phonemic system has been learned.

As I noted in the previous chapter, there are good reasons to believe that the early use of print actually has deleterious effects on speech production. The basic problem is that speech consists of patterns in time whereas print consists of patterns in space. The only temporal speech feature which is encoded in print is that of sequence, and even then the left-to-right, top-to-bottom convention is an arbitrary one that must be learned by the child. There is nothing in written language to provide information about the relative durations of sounds, syllables, words, or pauses or about the intonation patterns of speech. Remember that all written languages are an imperfect attempt to reencode, in spatial form, an already acquired spoken language. By all means let the child gain familiarity with the symbols and order of written language but do not teach speech as a reencoding of print. If you do so, you virtually guarantee the choppy, arhythmic, monotone speech that is so frequently encountered among deaf children.

total communication

Nor should you expect help in the acquisition of motor speech skills from the addition of signs to the speech input. The purpose of all of the speech supplements—cues, print, and sign—is to facilitate linguistic and communicative development. They have no direct role to play in speech development.

input and feedback channels

After so many discouraging comments, you might well ask whether there are *any* adequate ways for hearing-impaired children to receive information about their own and others' speech. The answer is yes.

1. *Hearing* With proper amplification and good auditory management, there are very few hearing-impaired children who gain no information from hearing. Even among those with profound hearing losses, well over half can perceive the rhythm and intonation of speech auditorily. (See Chapter Eight.)

2. *Hearing and Vision* The addition of vision to hearing provides information that may not be available from either alone. A good example is the feature of voicing of consonants.

3. *Vision* Vision, by itself, is a poor source of input information, and it requires a mirror for feedback. Nevertheless, it can be used to help teach the configurations, positions, and movements of the jaw, tongue, and lips.

4. *Touch* Children can feel, with their hands, vibrations of the oral and nasal cavities and the direction, rate, and time pattern of air flow. To a certain extent they can also feel tongue position and configuration by manual exploration.

5. *Instrumental Aids* There are many ways in which information about speech can be converted into signals that can be seen or felt by a hearing-impaired child. Among very simple devices is the feather, which can reveal the direction, rate, and time pattern of air flow. Among the most complex is the Speech Spectrum Display which analyzes speech and shows an instantaneous spectrogram on a television screen.

6. *Description* Finally there is you, the teacher, who can if necessary tell the children how to produce a particular sound, and then serve as their ears, telling them about the accuracy of their production.

Treat the foregoing list as a system of priorities. If the child can perceive and imitate by hearing alone, this is the technique of choice. If not, try adding vision. If this still does not work, try adding touch and so on. Ultimately, the children will retain and control their new skills by means of internal sensory feedback, supplemented by whatever hearing they have. Your task is to find the means for them to learn the patterns of speech in the first place. This requires access to the motor-acoustic symbols of speech itself—not the substitution of manual or written symbols.

graded sequence

I referred earlier to the need, in an output-centered approach, for a carefully graded scheme of development that recognizes the child's need for mastery of all necessary subskills before tackling a new skill. Such a scheme has been developed by Ling and is described at length in his book, *Speech and the Hearing Impaired Child—Theory and Practice,* first published in 1976. Ling's approach is based on exhaustive review of the educational and research literature and on extensive practical experience. His book, which was the first of its kind to be published in over 40 years, had a major impact on educators of the deaf, most of whom were dissatisfied with existing, empirically based approaches.

It is important to recognize that Ling did not develop new techniques for speech teaching. His contribution was to take the results of several decades of research in speech and hearing science and apply them to the development of an approach that is systematically organized, scientifically and educationally valid, and demonstrably effective. The influence of Ling's work on the present chapter is hereby acknowledged.

○ OBJECTIVES

If this phase of management is successful, the child will

1. Use normal patterns of breathing for speech production.
2. Use normal (or at least effective) patterns of voicing.
3. Use normal (or at least effective) patterns of rhythm and intonation.
4. Generate a normal (or at least effective) vowel system.
5. Generate a normal (or at least effective) consonant system.
6. Combine speech sounds in a normal (or at least effective) way.
7. Incorporate these motor speech skills into expressive language behavior.

general

Before discussing the realization of these objectives I need to discuss, in general terms, how one elicits, reinforces, and modifies speech behavior.

The first requirement is a comfortable atmosphere. Nothing is more likely to inhibit speech output (even in normally hearing adults) than tension, frustration, embarrassment, and mistrust. You must establish rapport with the children, they must enjoy interacting with you and even more importantly, you must enjoy interacting with them.

Within a comfortable environment, and during enjoyable, dynamic activities, the chances are that children will vocalize spontaneously. Beyond this, the only way to elicit speech is by imitation. Make sure that the children have the concept of imitation and if you need to establish imitative routines, do so first with nonspeech activities. Let imitation be a two-way street—take turns, in order that the children can discover the pleasure of control that eventually will come through speech. When first working on imitation of speech, the children must perceive your utterances and their own utterances through the same modality. The modality of choice is obviously hearing but when you are dealing with features to which a child has no auditory access, you must use alternatives. Let me stress again that in each case, the children must perceive your utterances and their utterances in the same way. If they see your speech movements, they must see their own for comparison. If they feel your speech postures, they must feel their own, and so on. This is a very basic point that is frequently overlooked in imitative speech work. Only when children have established the necessary associations, should you expect them to perceive your input and their output through different modalities.

As you work on imitative activities, establish some signal, such as the passing of a microphone, to indicate, "Do what I did." This will be very important in later stages of speech work when the child will need to distinguish between "Do what I did" and "Respond to what I said."

You can reinforce desirable speech outputs socially—with approval or disapproval—and tangibly—with candy, favorite games, and so on. Tangible reinforcement should not be your primary tool, but it can be a useful supplement and adds variety.

The best reinforcement is undoubtedly that which comes from the discovery of control. The auditory child will work hard on speech development, just for the reward of controlling his or her own acoustic input. The nonauditory child may similarly be motivated by the control of a visual input if you use flashing lights or moving toys controlled either electronically or through another person. (For example, you start the train when the child says, "Go.") The most powerful reinforcer is the control of other people. Once the child discovers that speech can make you do such things as stand up, sit down, start singing, go to sleep, wake up, jump in fright, start bouncing him or her on your knee, start scribbling, or draw a person, you should be able to elicit, sustain, and modify all the speech output you need.

The obvious question, however, is "How do you respond to incorrect output?" If the child fails to get positive reinforcement, or gets negative reinforcement (even a simple shaking of the head) for too great a proportion of the time, it is likely that speech output will be withheld rather than improved. Herein lies the need for the hierarchical, graded approach to which I referred previously. If you can organize your teaching so that the next step is always easy for the child by virtue of mastery of previous steps, your ratio of positive to negative reinforcement will remain high. If you find that the child is having difficulty with a new task, then you must back off and try to determine what intermediate steps are necessary to make the task less difficult.

This need for hierarchy has been considered in organizing the objectives listed earlier. The sequence is not a simple one, however. Breathing and voice production should be dealt with together, and the use of motor skills in expressive language should be pursued as soon as a skill is established. Note further that within each major level, there is a need for rational progression, but that complete mastery at one level is not necessary before moving on to the next. (Figure 10–1 illustrates this progression.)

developing speech breathing patterns

Speech is produced during exhalation, but the rate of air flow is much lower than that used in vegetative breathing, and most of the air flows through the mouth, rather than through the nose. Inhalation usually occurs at the end of a sentence and is faster than that used in vegetative breathing. If it is necessary to inhale within a sentence, we choose some point at which the brief pause will not interfere with syntactic structure.

Both normally hearing and hearing-impaired children use normal speech breathing patterns during the reflexive stages of vocalization and babbling but without intervention, the speech output of the hearing-impaired child is likely to stop. When you try to restart it, at a later date, the breathing patterns may well be abnormal—especially if you must use nonauditory teaching techniques. Typical errors include excessive air flow, excessive nasal air flow, frequent inhalations at inappropriate places, and the use of glottal stops to conserve air. What the child is trying to do is to superimpose speech onto vegetative breathing patterns. By early intervention we hope to capitalize on, and reinforce, the child's reflexive speech breathing

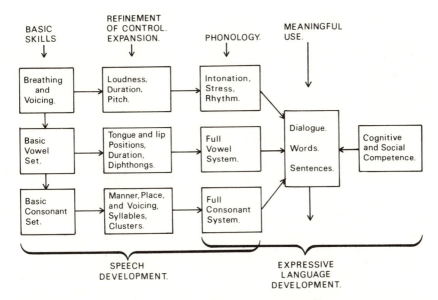

BASIC SKILLS ↓

REFINEMENT OF CONTROL. EXPANSION. ↓

PHONOLOGY. ↓

MEANINGFUL USE. ↓

| Breathing and Voicing. | Loudness, Duration, Pitch. | Intonation, Stress, Rhythm. |

| Basic Vowel Set. | Tongue and lip Positions, Duration, Diphthongs. | Full Vowel System. |

| Basic Consonant Set. | Manner, Place, and Voicing, Syllables, Clusters. | Full Consonant System. |

Dialogue. Words. Sentences.

Cognitive and Social Competence.

SPEECH DEVELOPMENT.

EXPRESSIVE LANGUAGE DEVELOPMENT.

FIGURE 10–1 A scheme for speech development. The child progresses from gross control of motor skills, through fine control, through the establishment of phonological patterns to the meaningful use of vocabulary and prosody. Note that progress must be made simultaneously in the three major areas—breath and voice control, vowel production, and consonant production. Note also that these three aspects of speech must be practiced together, so that they can be controlled independently of one another.

The information on the right of this figure has been included to emphasize that the motor skills of speech are acquired, not for their own sake, but for the role they will play in expressive language function. It is not meant to imply that full control of phonology must be established before speech is used meaningfully. Obviously the emerging speech skills must be capitalized on for communication as soon as possible.

patterns. If it is too late for this, then you must take whatever advantage you can of the child's auditory capacity. If he can hear the rhythm and intonation of speech, he will be constrained to use normal speech breathing in order to imitate your utterances. Late intervention with a nonauditory child poses serious problems. My suggestions are: use long utterances, and require their production on one breath; avoid tension or anxiety; play games that help the child gain conscious control of the breathing apparatus.

On this last point—breathing exercises—you must be very cautious. There is no clear evidence that such activities as blowing bubbles or blowing cotton balls with a straw produce results of direct relevance to speech production. It is true that there are some similarities of breathing pattern, but there are also some differences. Look on these activities as ways to exercise control of the breathing mechanism, not as ways of establishing basic speech postures.

developing voicing patterns

Voicing occurs when air escapes between closed vocal folds under certain conditions of subglottal pressure (that is, pressure in the lungs) and vocal fold tension. The resulting sound is a complex tone that, under normal conditions, meets the following criteria:

1. The fundamental frequency can be varied by the talker to produce patterns of intonation. This is done primarily by changing the tension of the vocal folds.
2. There is a minimum of aperiodic noise (breathiness). This is because the air flow is completely stopped by the vocal folds during at least 50 percent of the vibration cycle.
3. There is a high concentration of energy in the higher harmonics, making it possible to stimulate the higher frequency resonances of the air in the vocal tract. This again is due to the fact that the vocal folds open for only a small fraction of the vibration cycle.

Normal patterns of voicing, like the breathing patterns to which they are intimately related, appear in the reflexive vocalizations of children, regardless of their hearing status. The hearing-impaired child who learns speech late, and nonauditorily, is likely to exhibit a variety of voice problems. These include

1. Excessive vocal fold tension, requiring excessive subglottal pressure, and producing a high fundamental frequency.
2. Inadequate range of vocal fold tensions, leading to absence of intonation.
3. Incomplete closure of vocal folds, leading to excessive air flow, breathiness, and poorly defined vocal tract resonances.
4. Insufficient energy in the higher harmonics for adequate stimulation of those vocal tract resonances that encode articulatory information.
5. Abnormal postures of the supralaryngeal structures that change the spectrum to produce a nasal, or reedy, voice quality.

Voicing that exhibits these errors is neither pleasant nor effective.

To ensure good voicing patterns you should capitalize on and reinforce spontaneous vocalization; use audition as the modality of choice for input and feedback during imitative behavior; encourage the imitation of long utterances; and maintain a relaxed teaching atmosphere.

For the nonauditory child, use visual input and feedback (for example a voice-activated light or toy [see Figure 8–3]) and/or tactile input and feedback. In the latter case, the tactile sensation may be experienced directly by touching the face or indirectly by using an amplifier whose output is connected to a mechanical vibrator. As soon as possible, however, the child must learn to function independently of these aids.

Once conscious control of voicing has been obtained, you should aim for simultaneous and independent control of loudness, duration, pitch, and vocal tract configuration. This last carries you to the next phonetic level, which is the development of a vowel system.

Note that the nonauditory child can perceive the presence, duration, and loudness of voicing through the sense of touch. This modality cannot, however, be used to perceive pitch. If the child is to acquire control of this feature, you must use either instrumental aids (that is, visible pitch indicators) or descriptive input and feedback, indicating what you want—verbally or with hand positions—and saying whether the child got it right. Once pitch control is established, it can be maintained with internal sensory feedback.

developing rhythm and intonation patterns

English is normally spoken at a rate of four or five syllables per second, the durations of individual syllables varying widely according to their phonemic content and their syntactic and semantic roles. Each sentence contains one or more key words that carry a primary stress, and these stresses occur at approximately equal time intervals. Pauses are used to mark syntactic boundaries, for emphasis, or for inhalation. Inhalation occurs only when the resulting pause is syntactically and semantically appropriate. Sentences are characterized by a fairly steady average pitch and terminated by a pitch fall. Pitch changes above or below the average, are used along with increases of duration and (to a lesser extent) loudness to mark stresses and thus clarify the syntactic structure and the intended meaning. The termination of a sentence with a pitch rise indicates that the thought is not complete and is often used in questions to distinguish them from statements or to elicit a response.

Normally hearing children acquire the rhythmic and intonational properties of their language at a very early age—long before they have mastered the vowel and consonant system. Unlike breathing and voicing patterns, however, rhythm and intonation are not reflexive but purposeful—learned, by means of hearing, through imitation.

Hearing-impaired children, taught late and nonauditorily, often exhibit all or some of the following errors:

1. Very low rate (for example one syllable per second or less).

2. Failure to differentiate syllable durations.

3. Introduction of pauses at syntactically inappropriate places (sometimes after each word or syllable).

4. Absence of terminal fall.

5. Erratic changes of pitch that confuse the listener as to syntactic structure and the location of stress.

You should note that all children with severe hearing losses, and at least 50 percent of children with profound hearing losses, can perceive rhythm and intonation by hearing. There are two reasons for this: Information on rhythm and intonation is available in all parts of the speech spectrum (unlike information on place of articulation, which is concentrated in the higher frequencies); and the perception of speech rhythm and intonation does not require fine discrimination.

The implication is that *an input-centered, global, auditory approach should produce normal patterns of rhythm and intonation in the spoken language output of all but a small minority of hearing-impaired children.*

It is my belief that those children who lack the auditory capacity for the perception of intonation cannot be expected to acquire *normal* rhythm and intonation in their own speech. There is no reason, however, why they should not produce *effective* rhythm and intonation patterns.

By their very nature, rhythm and intonation are phonological speech features. There is, however, much that can be done at a phonetic level to facilitate their acquisition. I have already referred to the development of conscious control of duration, pitch, and loudness when working on breathing and voicing patterns. When you start to use syllable strings, you can make these follow the rules of sentences—lengthening the final syllable and allowing it to carry a pitch fall. You can also shift the stress from syllable to syllable, and you can require that the child work up to a syllable rate approximating that of normal speech.

Your own language input should have normal rhythm and intonation patterns. This sounds simple, but I am constantly amazed by the number of teachers who distort these speech features when talking to hearing-impaired children. The most common error is the omission of a terminal fall, presumably in an attempt to elicit repetition. This strategy, of course, presupposes the existence of the very skills you hope to teach, and at the same time gives the child a misleading model. The second most common error is for the teacher to use the rhythmic and intonational patterns that are common in the speech of hearing-impaired children. This seems to be an instinctive attempt to facilitate comprehension by adopting the listener's speech code. If you are in doubt about the normalcy of your own input, make tape recordings, and listen to yourself, or ask someone else to observe you.

At a very early stage of phonological development, the child should acquire a repertoire of simple utterances in which intonation is the primary carrier of information. Examples are "Uh, oh!" for a minor accident; "Uh, uh!" with headshaking for negation plus warning; "Wow!" for a pleasant surprise; and "Oh! No!" for an unpleasant surprise. You can use these frequently, in all kinds of situations, and with exaggerated intonation contours. Unless the child is nonauditory, he or she will learn them by imitation.

developing a vowel system

Voicing produces a complex sound that is rich in harmonics. As the sound passes through the vocal tract, the relative strengths of these harmonics are modified. What emerges from the lips carries not only the original characteristics of voicing but also the acoustical characteristics of the cavities of the mouth and throat. This second set of characteristics appears as concentrations of energy, known as *formants,* whose frequencies can be changed by movements of the jaw, tongue, and lips. In this way, articulatory information is carried from the talker's mouth to the listener's ears.

The formants are numbered, starting at the lowest frequency, and in an adult male, have the following average frequencies:

First formant (F1)   500 Hz

Second formant (F2)   1500 Hz

Third formant (F3)   2500 Hz and so on.

Variations of these formant frequencies produce identifiably different vowel qualities. By raising and lowering the tongue and jaw, we can change the value of F1 over a range from about 300 Hz to about 900 Hz. With the tongue in a raised position we can, by moving it backwards and forwards, change the value of F2 over a range from about 1000 Hz to about 3000 Hz. I cannot stress too strongly that the tongue is responsible for vowel articulation. The lips simply emphasize and exaggerate the acoustical changes produced by the tongue. Lip movements, however, are not essential, and lip movement alone cannot be used to produce an effective vowel system.

In any given language, six or seven vocal tract configurations are selected as the basis of a vowel system. This system can then be expanded by introducing long and short versions of each vowel, nasal and nonnasal versions (in French, for example), or by combining pairs of vowels to make diphthongs. Under normal circumstances the vowel system is learned through hearing, but once acquired, it may be sustained by internal sensory feedback.

Typical vowel errors in the speech of hearing-impaired children include

1. Inadequate range of tongue movements and hence of formant changes.

2. Failure to contrast long and short vowels.

3. Omission of one component of diphthongs.
4. Nasalization of all vowels.

Quite simply, the hearing-impaired child tends to reproduce the visible aspects of vowel articulation (that is lip and jaw movements) much more accurately than the invisible aspects (tongue and velum movements and duration). Unfortunately, the visible aspects, though useful for vowel perception, are relatively useless for learning vowel production.

All children with severe hearing losses, and many with profound hearing losses, should be able to learn the complete vowel system by imitation, using the sense of hearing. You can improve the audibility of the formants by placing vowels in the context of bilabial consonants (for example, "Baaah!" "Boo!" "Peep" and so on). It seems that the neural mechanisms of hearing may be predisposed to respond to the rapid changes of formant frequency that occur at the junctions between vowels and consonants. You can further improve the audibility of the second formant (F2) for some children, by using whispered speech. Whispering reduces the strength of F1 and may be useful for children who can hear F2, but not in the presence of F1. If children are unable to imitate vowels by hearing alone, then try vision, but remember that it is your tongue position they must see and copy—not just your lip and jaw positions. If necessary, you may allow them to feel the position and configuration of your tongue and then feel their own for comparison. Some instrumental speech training aids reveal formant frequencies through visible or tactile displays. There are, however, very few research findings to indicate their potential role with very young children. If you use such aids, do so with caution. Your final option is to tell the child how to position his or her tongue—perhaps using models, drawings, or hand positions.

The most easily acquired vowel is /a/, since this involves a lowered jaw and relaxed tongue.* Once /a/ is mastered, you should proceed to the high vowels /u/ and /i/. These three vowels form the corners of a *vowel triangle* that can now be expanded by adding three intermediate vowels, by contrasting long and short vowels, and by adding diphthongs. (See Figure 10–2).

Note that, once the vowels /a/, /u/ and /i/ have been mastered, you should begin work on the next level of speech development—consonant articulation.

As the child's vowel system expands you must require

1. Variations of loudness, duration, and pitch, independently of tongue, jaw, and lip configuration.
2. Production of the vowel without nasal resonance.
3. Production of the vowel in rapid syllable strings, (for example, /babababa b/).

*I.p.a. symbols will be used throughout this chapter.

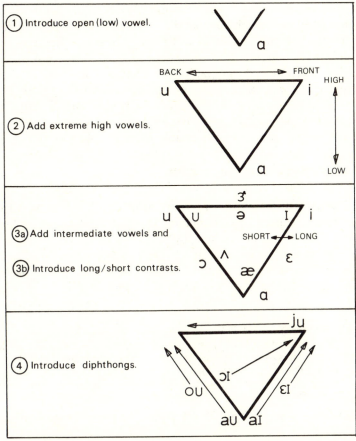

FIGURE 10–2 A developmental sequence for vowels. Note that each vowel must be practiced in combination with various consonants.

4. Alternation with other vowels in syllable strings, (for example, /babibabib/).

5. Incorporation into everyday vocabulary. (See Figure 10–4 for examples.)

This stage of your work requires sensitivity to regional differences of accent or dialect. There is no reason, for example, why a teacher in Louisiana should teach her children the vowel system of Bostonian English.

Before leaving the topic of vowel production, I must make one final comment about imitation. *Before* a vowel system has been learned, the only means by which a child can directly imitate vowels is by hearing. Quite simply, the child tries to match your acoustic patterns on the basis of previously acquired knowledge about the relationship between speech sound and speech movement. *After* a vowel system is established, children do not imitate in the same way. They identify and produce. If, for example, you say

/i/, the children recognize this as belonging to a category within their vowel system and produce their own example of a vowel belonging to that category. This kind of imitation does not require hearing. The vowel can be identified from lip configuration alone, if necessary. This means that you can employ direct imitation during language development even with nonauditory children, *providing they have first established a vowel system.* Note, however, that this comment applies only to stressed vowels and diphthongs. Unstressed vowels tend to lose their characteristic lip configurations, and the consonants are not uniquely identifiable from visual clues alone.

developing a consonant system

Connected speech may be thought of as a long stream of vowels, periodically interrupted by consonants. The best analogy I can think of is the creation of a string of sausages by periodically pinching and twisting a long tube filled with sausage meat.

Consonants are usually brief and involve complete or partial interruption of air flow through the mouth. They may be classified in several ways:

1. By manner of articulation:
   Stops and affricates—These involve complete stoppage of air flow. Continuants—These involve partial stoppage of air flow. a) Nasals—The air flow is redirected through the nose. b) Vowellike consonants—The articulators slide to or from a vowel configuration. c) Fricatives—Turbulent airflow is produced at a narrow constriction.

2. By place of articulation. This describes the place of maximum vocal tract constriction, which may be:
   At the lips (bilabial)
   Between lower lips and upper teeth (labiodental)
   Between tongue and upper teeth (linguadental)
   Between tongue and gum ridge (lingua-alveolar)
   Between tongue and hard palate (linguapalatal)
   Between tongue and soft palate (linguavelar)
   At the glottis (glottal)

3. By voicing. The stops, affricates, and fricatives mostly come in two versions:
   Voiced
   Voiceless

For ease of reference this consonant classification system is presented in Figure 10–3.

The consonant system is normally learned through the sense of hearing, but its control is sustained mainly by internal sensory feedback—we remember how the consonants should feel, rather than how they should sound. A child's ability to hear consonant information varies not only with degree of

		STOPS and AFFRICATES				CONTINUANTS					
		STOPS		AFFRICATES		NASALS		QUASI-VOWELS		FRICATIVES	
	BILABIAL	b	p			m		w			hw
	LABIODENTAL									v	f
	LINGUADENTAL									ð	θ
	LINGUA-ALVEOLAR	d	t			n		j		z	s
	LINGUAPALATAL			dʒ	tʃ			r		ʒ	ʃ
	LINGUAVELAR	g	k			ŋ					
	GLOTTAL	ʔ									h
		VOICED	VOICE-LESS	VOICED	VOICE-LESS	VOICED	VOICE-LESS	VOICED	VOICE-LESS	VOICED	VOICE-LESS

PLACE OF ARTICULATION (left side label)

VOICING

FIGURE 10–3 English consonants classified according to manner of articulation, place of articulation, and voicing. Note: a) The contrast between /w/ and /hw/ is seldom used and need not be taught to deaf children; b) The glottal stop /ʔ/ is not a contrastive phoneme but is often substituted for /t/; c) The aspirate /h/ does not have a specific place of articulation. It normally takes on the articulatory configuration of the following vowel; d) In developing a system of consonants, manner contrasts should be taught first using the bilabial consonants. Place of articulation contrasts can then be introduced, followed by voiced-voiceless contrasts.

hearing loss but also with consonant feature. Children with moderate hearing losses, for example, should have full access, through hearing, to all consonant features. Children with severe hearing losses have difficulty hearing place of articulation but should be able to hear manner and voicing. Children with profound hearing losses need a combination of vision and hearing to perceive place and voicing contrasts but should be able to hear many manner contrasts. Totally deaf children can perceive some information about place of articulation visually but need indirect techniques to perceive the remaining features. Some of these techniques include observing the effects of the breathstream on candle flames, feathers, or tissue; feeling surface vibrations of the face and nose; feeling air flow from the mouth; using instrumental aids such as voicing, nasality, and sibilant indicators; or describing articulatory postures.

The development of a consonant system should follow a logical scheme, beginning with the easier skills and progressing to the more difficult ones. Labial consonants offer lots of visual and auditory information and provide a way of distinguishing the major manner categories. You might therefore begin with

a bilabial stop	—/b/ or /p/
a bilabial nasal continuant	—/m/
a bilabial nonnasal continuant	—/w/
a labiodental fricative	—/f/ or /v/

These should be produced

1. In association with each of the three primary vowels—/a/, /u/ or /i/.
2. In syllable strings (for example, /bababa/).
3. In syllable strings alternated with other consonants (for example, /bamabama/).
4. At a syllable rate approximating that of normal conversational speech.
5. Without affecting voice loudness or pitch.
6. At the ends of syllable strings as well as at the beginning (for example, /bababab/).
   (Note that the effect of a final /w/ is to diphthongize the previous vowel, for example, /wawawaʊ/.)

As soon as the children have comfortable control of these consonants, they should incorporate them into spoken language. For example,

/p/ or /b/ →ball, bye bye, bib, up, and so on
/m/ →me, Mommy, milk, warm, home, and so on
/w/ →walk, wash, where, wow, and so on
/v/ or /f/ →fall, face, knife, laugh.

Each of the major categories should be expanded by moving back in terms of place of articulation, that is, following the columns of Figure 10–3 (omitting, for the time being, the affricates).

When manner and place contrasts have been consolidated, you can introduce the fricative-affricate contrast (shoe-chew), and finally the voiced-voiceless contrasts. At each level you must ensure that the consonants are produced with a minimum of effort; in rapid syllable strings; independently of loudness, pitch, or vowel context; and in communicative speech.

developing phoneme combinations

It is tempting to think of speech sounds as separate entities that can be strung together like beads. This model may be accurate at some internal level of representation, either before speech is generated or after it has been recognized, but it cannot be applied to the motor-acoustic events of speech itself. At least six independent sets of muscles are involved in speech production—those of breathing, the larynx, the velum, the tongue, the jaw, and the lips. A speech sound may be thought of as a cluster of six target conditions. In connected speech, each muscle set is in a constant state of change from one target condition to another. The way a particular target is approached, held, and left depends not only on the particular sound but also on what came before and what comes after. If you need a model, you should think of six multicolored strands being braided to form a rope with a sequential pattern.

The implication of the foregoing is that hearing-impaired children must learn not only the target conditions for each vowel and consonant but also the appropriate movements to, from, and between these conditions. It is for this reason that they must practise consonants in combination with several vowels, vowels in combination with several consonants, consonants in rapid syllable strings (both repeated and alternated with other consonants), and consonants in initial, medial, and final positions. The child who can only say /ba/ cannot be said to have mastered the consonant /b/.

A special set of problems is encountered when consonants must be combined in clusters. Such combinations generally require much more rapid and accurately coordinated movements than are found in consonant-vowel combinations. Sometimes the target conditions are changed (as in the devoicing of /l/ in *pl*ay); sometimes the consonants are articulated sequentially (as in *st*ick); sometimes they are articulated simultaneously (as in *bl*ow).

Nasal-stop blends (as in ju*mp*) require precise timing of velar movements, and when a stop comes first, it is released, not through the mouth, but through the nose (as in a*t n*ine). When two stops occur together, the release of the first one is usually omitted (as in cu*pc*ake), and when two identical consonants are combined, they are usually made into one consonant of longer duration (as in so*me mi*ce).

You cannot, therefore, rest on your laurels once the child has mastered the consonant system. You must teach consonant combinations as though they were a whole new group of sounds. If he or she cannot imitate them using auditory input and feedback, you must work from existing skills using, for example, strings of CVC syllables such as

noʊs/→noʊs/noʊ/→*snow*

The developmental sequence recommended by Ling is as follows:

1. Word Initial Blends
   Sequential Blends
   a) Using two organs, for example, /sm/
   b) Using the same organ, for example, /sk/
   Simultaneous Blends
   a) Using two organs, for example, /bl/
   b) Using the same organ, for example, /dr/
   Triple Blends, for example, /skr/

2. Word Final Blends
   Continuant first
   a) Continuant-continuant blends, for example, /fs/
   b) Continuant-stop blends, for example, /ft/

Stop first
a) Stop-continuant blends, for example, /ts/
b) Stop-stop blends, for example, /pt/
Triple blends, for example, /fts/

For a detailed discussion of this and other aspects of speech development, I must refer you to Ling's own (1976) publication.

incorporating speech skills into expressive language

The biggest danger in this phase of your work is that of becoming so engrossed in the motor skills of speech that they become an end in themselves. Remember always that speech only exists as a medium for the externalization and exchange of linguistically encoded thoughts. Without language there is no speech—only noises.

At each level of skill development you must contrive ways of helping the children discover that their new skills can be used to increase the effectiveness of verbal language output. At first they must learn that vocalization controls people. Next they must learn that simple vocalization is not enough. You must require them to produce utterances of sentence length —with at least one identifiable word. At first only the central vowel need be accurate, but as the children master more and more sounds in an ever increasing vocabulary, you must require their incorporation into sentences. With early intervention, a carefully graded hierarchy of skills, spontaneous interaction, a clear concept of the child's level of attainment, and a relaxed attitude, this can be done without undue interruption of the communication process and without creating speech anxiety.

○ WHAT TO EXPECT

With early and skillful intervention, the neurologically intact, hearing-impaired child, in a stimulating and supportive home environment, should be able to acquire effective speech skills regardless of the degree of hearing loss. That is to say, his or her speech patterns should be consistent, differentiated, and intelligible to all family members and most strangers. To the extent that the child has the auditory capacity for perception and control, you should expect not just effective patterns but normal patterns. For many children with profound losses, expect normal patterns of breathing, rhythm, and intonation, and perhaps normal patterns of vowel articulation and manner and voicing of consonants. For children with severe losses, you should certainly expect normal patterns of vowel articulation, and manner and voicing of consonants, and adequate place of articulation of consonants.

Much will depend, of course, on the age at which intervention began, the suitability of the hearing aids, and the amount of time devoted to speech development. This last point raises one of the more serious issues in deaf education. In the face of a multiplicity of developmental needs, how much priority should be given to the mastery of the motor skills of speech? There are educators who unhesitatingly make speech acquisition (or more correctly—spoken language acquisition) a major goal, to be pursued, if necessary, at the expense of other needs. At the opposite end of the spectrum are educators who place social, emotional, cognitive, and linguistic development ahead of speech development and will only contemplate work on the last to the extent that it does not interfere with the others.

One of the good things about early intervention is that it provides access to the child at a time when speech development can be pursued as a natural component of an overall approach that addresses all major needs. In the hands of a competent teacher, and with highly motivated and well-adjusted parents, there need be no conflict.

If you are working with a child whose progress is slow, or who appears to be developing negative emotional reactions to speech, you must try to determine the cause. One possibility is that you are moving too quickly. Do not expect the child to master a new skill until all the subskills are thoroughly mastered. Another possibility is that there is too much pressure to perform from the parents. If you are going to be aggressive about the early acquisition of speech skills, I believe this is one aspect of management that you must handle in one-to-one instruction. Instruct and advise the parents on ways to use and consolidate the child's newly acquired phonological skills, but do not involve them directly in phonetic skill development. A third possibility is that the child just cannot master certain speech skills. This may be due to an anatomical problem, such as an inability to close the velopharyngeal port. Alternatively, it may be the result of a neurological problem that interferes with development of adequate control of the speech musculature, memory for patterns of motor behavior, or establishment of associations between sensory input, motor output, and internal phonological or linguistic schemata. If you believe you have learned the cause of your difficulties, use this information, together with your experience and knowledge, to determine whether the child requires different teaching strategies, more or less pressure to progress, more intensive parent counselling, or access to an alternative expressive modality, such as sign language.

○ DELIVERY

Developmental speech work must be done as a one-to-one activity. It can be integrated into a parent guidance program, in which the child is seen with his parents for one or two hours a week, or it can be built into a nursery or preschool program during which the child leaves the group for 20 or 30 minutes per day. This time must be shared between speech development, language development, and auditory development. This is not to suggest, however, that these activities compete with each other. On the contrary, in the hands of a first class teacher, they support and reinforce each other.

Just as we have seen audiologists becoming increasingly involved in auditory aspects of management, so we have seen speech pathologists becoming increasingly involved in speech aspects of management. My reaction to these developments is the same. The basic training of a speech pathologist is not an adequate preparation for this kind of work. By the same token, however, neither is the basic training of a teacher of the deaf. The one knows too little about deafness; the other knows too little about speech. Whatever your basic disciplinary background, you must prepare yourself for this kind of work by additional training, study, and supervised practice.

○ EVALUATION

The best tool for speech evaluation is undoubtedly the human ear. It is, therefore, up to you to listen to the child's speech and determine how well various objectives have been met. As you do so, observe the following words of caution:

1. Listen to the sounds the child actually makes, resisting the natural tendency to fill in missing information or to transform sounds from what they are into what you know they are supposed to be.

2. Do no be satisfied that the child's vocabulary is intelligible to you and the family. Find out whether it is intelligible to strangers.

3. Do not be satisfied that certain sounds are present; ask also whether they provide contrasts of meaning (for example, *my* and *bye*) independently of context.

4. Do not be satisfied with speech sounds that are used only on demand; ask also whether they are used in spontaneous communication.

5. Check your observations against those of a qualified and independent observer. *It takes years of listening and study to develop truly objective listening skills that permit identification of speech errors and diagnosis of their cause.*

6. Whenever feasible, support your judgments with physical measurements. Parameters such as syllable rate and fundamental frequency are not difficult to measure with modern speech analysis equipment.

The objectives listed earlier in this chapter provide a general outline for evaluation, but each needs expanding.

Breathing Ask about inhalation; the rate, duration, and direction of expiration; and the use of glottal stops.

Voicing Ask whether voicing is under voluntary control and whether the parameters of loudness, duration, and pitch can be varied at will. In spontaneous speech, ask about the volume, pitch, and quality of voice.

Timing Ask about syllable rate and variations of syllable duration. Ask also whether the speech flows together or whether it is interrupted by inappropriate pauses.

Intonation Ask whether sentence ends are marked by falling pitch and whether pitch variations are used to mark stress and emphasis.

Vowel System Ask whether the child contrasts high and low vowels, front and back vowels, short and long vowels, and pure vowels and diphthongs. Record his or her ability to produce each vowel, on demand, in various contexts, and in spoken language. (See Figure 10–4 for a suggested evaluation form.)

Consonant System Ask whether the child contrasts consonants on the basis of manner of articulation, place of articulation, and voicing. Record his or her ability to produce each consonant on demand, in various contexts, and in spoken language. (See Figure 10–5 for a suggested evaluation form.)

Consonant Blends Ask whether the child can combine two or three consonants into a single blend, in both word initial and word final position.

FIGURE 10–4   An evaluation form for vowels. Mastery of a specific skill can be indicated by a check. Allowances must be made for regional accents, to which vowels are particularly susceptible.

	Long vowels						Short vowels					Diphthongs						
	ɑ	u	i	ɔ	ɛ	ɜ	æ	ʊ	ɪ	ʌ	ə	aʊ	aɪ	oʊ	ɪə	ɔɪ	ju	
In isolation																		⎫
Varying length																		Phonetic
Varying loudness																		level
Varying pitch																		
In syllable strings																		⎭
In words																		⎫
Sample words:	arm,car,hot	shoe,two	eat,teeth,Mommy	fall,ball	bed,yes	girl,dirty	Daddy,bang	look,cookie	hit,milk	up,thumb	today,a,water	down,out,house	cry,mine,I	no,soap	baby,wave	boy,noisy	new	Phonological level

	Stops & Affricates								Nasals			Quasi-vowels				Fricatives									
	p	b	t	d	k	g	tʃ	dʒ	m	n	ŋ	w	j	r	l	hw	f	v	θ	ð	s	z	ʃ	ʒ	h
In isolation																									
Single syllable																treat as /w/									
Initial and final											░	░											░	░	
Syllable strings																									
With each vowel																									
Alternating consonants																░									
In words																░									
Sample words:	up,push	byebye,ball	hat,teeth	down,bed	sick,kiss	good,big	chair,catch	juice,bridge	Mommy,home	no,run	ring,finger	one,window,why	you,yoyo	run,carry	light,pull	fall,half	vest,love	thumb,tooth	the,breathe	see,dress	zipper,cars	shoe,wash	treasure	hand,help	

Phonetic level (top six rows); Phonological level (In words / Sample words).

FIGURE 10–5 An evaluation form for consonants. Mastery of a specific skill can be indicated by a check. Note that for many speakers, the consonant /r/ does not occur in word-final position. When it does occur, the tendency is to modify the preceding vowel by retroflexion of the tongue tip. Note also that voiced-voiceless contrasts can be ignored in the early stages of speech development.

FIGURE 10–6 An evaluation form for word-initial consonant pairs. One check may be used to indicate mastery in syllables. A second check may be used to indicate mastery in words.

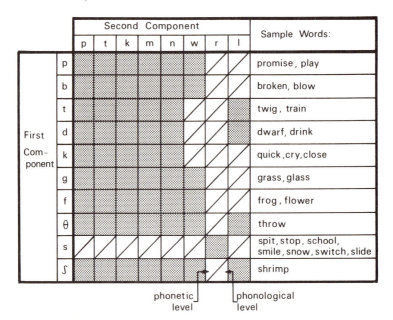

First Component	Second Component								Sample Words:
	p	t	k	m	n	w	r	l	
p									promise, play
b									broken, blow
t									twig, train
d									dwarf, drink
k									quick, cry, close
g									grass, glass
f									frog, flower
θ									throw
s									spit, stop, school, smile, snow, switch, slide
ʃ									shrimp

phonetic level / phonological level

168

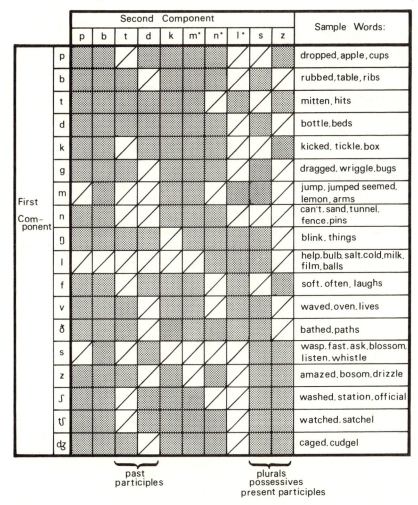

		Second Component									Sample Words:
		p	b	t	d	k	m*	n*	l*	s	z	
First Component	p											dropped, apple, cups
	b											rubbed, table, ribs
	t											mitten, hits
	d											bottle, beds
	k											kicked, tickle, box
	g											dragged, wriggle, bugs
	m											jump, jumped seemed, lemon, arms
	n											can't, sand, tunnel, fence, pins
	ŋ											blink, things
	l											help, bulb, salt, cold, milk, film, balls
	f											soft, often, laughs
	v											waved, oven, lives
	ð											bathed, paths
	s											wasp, fast, ask, blossom, listen, whistle
	z											amazed, bosom, drizzle
	ʃ											washed, station, official
	tʃ											watched, satchel
	dʒ											caged, cudgel

past participles   plurals possessives present participles

FIGURE 10–7 An evaluation form for word-final consonant pairs. One check may be used to indicate mastery in syllables. A second check may be used to indicate mastery in words. *Note that /m/, /n/, and /l/ often function as a syllable in this context.

Record his or her ability to produce each blend on demand and in spoken language. (See Figures 10–6 and 10–7 for suggested evaluation forms.)

Intelligibility Using tape recorded samples of conversational speech, determine the percentage of words correctly recognized by independent listeners. For the highest possible face validity, use listeners who are unfamiliar with the speech of hearing-impaired children. Make careful notes of the way the samples were obtained and the criteria for selecting listeners.

Approaches to speech instruction may be input-centered or output-centered, and they may be global or analytic. The appropriate balance depends on auditory capacity and on the particular speech skill being developed. Input and feedback channels include (in order of priority) audition, vision, touch, instrumental aids, and description. Cues, fingerspelling, sign, and print do not contribute to the acquisition of basic speech skills. Once a phonetic system has been established, however, these supplements can be useful in developing new vocabulary and correcting pronunciation.

The use of an output-centered approach requires a carefully graded, developmental scheme that permits the child to progress in small steps, consolidating essential subskills on the way. Such a scheme permits the child to experience a maximum of success and reduces anxiety and other negative reactions.

The proposed scheme is based on the work of Ling. The objectives are the establishment of breathing and voice patterns, a vowel system, a consonant system, and the skills of combining consonants. As soon as phonetic skills are established, they must be incorporated into vocabulary which is both meaningful and useful to the child.

Developmental speech work should be carried out by persons specially trained for this work. The parents' role should be that of encouraging and consolidating new speech skills.

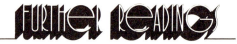

Daniel Ling's text *Speech and the Hearing Impaired Child* (A. G. Bell Association for the Deaf, Washington, D.C., 1976) offers both an exhaustive review of the literature and a carefully structured program of development. Other useful texts are Sir Alexander and Lady Ethel Ewing's *Teaching Deaf Children to Talk* (Manchester University Press, Manchester, U.K., 1964), Eleanor Vorce's *Teaching Speech to Deaf Children* (A. G. Bell Association for the Deaf, Washington, D. C., 1974) and Donald Calvert and Richard Silverman's *Speech and Deafness* (A. G. Bell Association for the Deaf, Washington, D.C., 1975). The chapters by Eleanor Vorce and Marjorie Magner in *Speech for the Deaf Child,* edited by L. E. Connor, (A. G. Bell Association for the Deaf, Washington, D.C., 1971) should also be included in your reading, although they both are concerned mainly with school-age children.

For a thorough introduction to speech science, I recommend F. D. Minifie, Thomas Hixon, and F. Williams' *Normal Aspects of Speech, Hearing and Language* (Prentice-Hall, Inc., Englewood Cliffs, N.J., 1973). William Tiffany and James Carrell's *Phonetics —Theory and Application* (McGraw-Hill, New York, 1977) should help replenish your knowledge of phonetics.

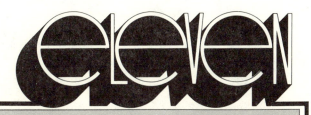

○ OBJECTIVES

○ PROCEDURES

coming to terms with feelings
learning about deafness
acquiring skills
making decisions

○ WHAT TO EXPECT

○ EVALUATION

○ SUMMARY

○ FURTHER READINGS

Parental management

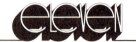

When the hearing-impaired child is below two and a half years of age, you cannot expect to influence his social, emotional, cognitive, and linguistic development except through his parents or their surrogates. Even at three or four years of age, when you can begin to exert direct influence, it is still the parents who have the most control over the child's environment—both physical and social. It follows that the success of an early intervention program depends largely on the success of its parental component. This is the foundation on which management must be built. I refer you to Chapter Five for a review of parental reactions and their influence on the development of the child.

○ OBJECTIVES

If this aspect of management is dealt with successfully, the parents will

1. Come to terms with their feelings.
2. Become knowledgeable about hearing impairment.
3. Provide an optimal learning environment for their child.
4. Be prepared to make major decisions affecting their child's future.

○ PROCEDURES

coming to terms with feelings

Maturation is a continuous process of accommodation to changes in our world and in ourselves. From time to time these changes are too sudden, too great, or too unwanted, and we cannot accommodate quickly enough. We then experience a sense of crisis and may require more outside support than is available through friends and family. At such times, an overriding feeling is that of loss. There may, in fact, be a real loss—as in the death of a loved one or the loss of a job. Alternatively, the loss may be more abstract—as in the loss of innocence that accompanies adolescence or the loss of a sense of immortality which often accompanies middle age. In all these crises, the true loss is an internal one. It is the loss of a secure world model that has become obsolete because of changed circumstances or increased awareness. Such is the situation of parents who have just learned that their child is deaf. (See Chapter Five.)

In your interactions with parents, you can offer some of the support they need while passing through the various stages of mourning. There are essentially three contexts:

1. Individual sessions in which your primary concern is parent education and instruction.
2. Individual sessions that are set aside for counselling.
3. Group sessions that offer the chance for mutual support among several parents.

A common feature of these contexts is that they provide a safe place in which parents can externalize, expose, and explore their feelings. Through your responses they can discover that it is not bad to be angry or to have feelings of rejection towards their child. They can discover that it is not unusual to feel overwhelmed or inadequate, and they can learn, at least intellectually, that they will survive and grow. They can discover that it is possible, indeed normal, to experience incompatible emotions and by sharing thoughts and feelings with other parents, they can begin to lose their sense of isolation.

When interacting with parents there are only a few positive things to remember:

DO • Listen when parents talk about their feelings. Save the instruction and opinion for later.

DO • Show that you are listening by occasional nods, "yeses," and brief summaries of what they have said (for example, "So you think the hearing aids sort of advertise the deafness?")

DO • Offer verbal expressions of feeling if the parents seem to have difficulty externalizing them (for example, "That must have made you very angry.")

DO • Answer questions directly and honestly when asked (for example, "No! Her speech will not sound normal.")

The list of negatives is somewhat longer:

DON'T • Deny the reality of the parents own feelings (for example, "Think how much worse it is for parents of mentally retarded children.")

DON'T • Imply that you are going to solve their problems by restoring the "normal" child they have lost.

DON'T • Try to impose on them your own opinions and ideologies.

DON'T • Overwhelm the parents with answers to questions they have not asked.

DON'T • Play on their guilt in order to get them to do what you believe to be good for the child.

DON'T • Respond negatively or judgmentally to honest expressions of feeling.

DON'T • Tell them you know how they feel.

Be careful to remain within the confines of your own expertise. Unless you are trained in counselling or psychotherapy, you should do nothing more than try to help otherwise well-adjusted people through a series of natural reactions to an unusually stressful situation. If the hearing-impaired child has had the misfortune to be born into a family where there are serious difficulties in coping with the everyday stresses of life, it is not your responsibility to try to deal with those difficulties. Refer the family to a suitably qualified individual.

One final word of caution. If you find yourself enjoying and encouraging the parents' emotional dependence, then you are in the wrong profession. You must help them stand on their own feet, not use them to satisfy some unmet need in yourself. Before you presume to interfere in the emotional lives of others, make sure that your own emotional house is in order.

learning about deafness

The curriculum for a program of parent education should include the material covered in Chapters One through Five of this book. You must, however, reduce it to its bare essentials and present it in terms appropriate to the parents with whom you are dealing. A list of topics that should be covered is given in Figure 11–1. These can be discussed incidentally during parent instruction and counselling, they can be handled more formally during individual or group parent meetings, or they can be explained in pamphlets and information sheets. (See, for example Appendix D.) A combination of these approaches is probably the most effective.

FIGURE 11–1 Suggested outline for a program of parent education

Child Development

Milestones
Concepts, words, sentences, and speech

Needs and Priorities

Love, acceptance, and respect
Exploration, problem solving, and testing
Playing with things, playing with people
Toys
Predictability, consistency, and limits
Discipline—defining who decides what

Hearing

Detection vs. interpretation
Role in language and speech development
Conductive, sensory, and neural mechanisms
Learning to hear

Hearing Impairment

What goes wrong and why
Conductive vs. sensorineural damage
Effects of degree of hearing loss
Possibilities for medicine and surgery
Need for hearing conservation
Interpreting audiograms and other hearing test results
Possibilities of auditory development

Hearing Aids

Function
Purpose
Types
Roles and limitations
Possibilities for the future

Education

Goals
History
Models and philosophies
Benefits and limitations of oral education
Benefits and limitations of manual communication
State and federal laws
Parents' rights and responsibilities

acquiring skills

Among the practical skills that the parents must acquire are

1. Monitoring hearing aids, identifying faults, effecting minor repairs, and cleaning earmolds.
2. Using play and the activities of daily living to stimulate and reinforce the child's
   development of cognitive and interactive skills.
3. Controlling the child's experience of sound so as to promote auditory development.
4. Controlling the child's experience of language so as to promote his or her own
   language development. (This requirement applies regardless of the particular
   modality being used for language.)
5. Developing strategies to encourage, sustain, and reinforce the child's speech
   output without creating tension or anxiety.

These skills can be taught during weekly sessions lasting perhaps one
hour each. You must, of course, have these skills yourself and be able to

demonstrate them to the parents with their own child. As they try to follow your lead, you must offer encouragement and constructive criticism.

There are several reasons for doing this work in the child's own home. This is probably the place where the child and parents will feel most comfortable; the objects being used will be familiar to the child; and you will have an opportunity to observe some of the practical constraints imposed by the home, the neighborhood, and other family members.

There may, however, be cogent reasons for having the parents come to a clinic or speech and hearing center. Teachers who spend several hours a week on the road are not using using their time and professional training in the most efficient, or cost effective, way; the atmosphere in a clinic may be less distracting and more businesslike than at home; and ready access can be had to such things as hearing aid repair facilities and video and audio tape recorders. In several centers where this type of work is undertaken, a compromise has been sought by building a model home or model apartment.

Some educators ask parents to set aside a fixed period of time each day for one-to-one interaction with the child. Into this time the bulk of the efforts at experiential, linguistic, and auditory stimulation are concentrated. Others favor a global approach in which parents are taught to interact more effectively with the child all day. It has been my experience that parents tend to fall into one of two major groups. In the first are parents who interact easily and spontaneously with their children and quickly grasp the principles underlying good habilitative management. Such parents provide their child with a warm, secure, and stimulating environment that has multiple learning opportunities and in which a special teaching session becomes redundant. In the second group are parents who are struggling to cope with a variety of demands, who have difficulty understanding the reasons behind what they are being asked to do, and who cannot see the world through a child's eyes. Such parents tend to leave their children to amuse themselves whenever possible and only interact out of necessity or crisis. For these parents, the imposition of a routine that includes a daily period of individual attention may be the only way of meeting the child's needs. As in all of this work, there is no single best method. You must remain sensitive to individual needs and be flexible in your approach.

making decisions

Through success in meeting the three previous objectives, the parents should acquire the confidence to make decisions. As they emerge from the mourning process, they will lose the feeling of impotence that it engenders and regain a sense of control. The educational component should provide them with factual information against which to evaluate choices, and the progress of their child should provide concrete evidence of their own abilities.

The parents will, of course, receive advice from relatives and from other professionals. When this occurs, they may turn to you for support or to confirm information previously given. Help them to define their goals and to evaluate their choices; remind them of the constraints under which they are working; but resist the temptation to make decisions for them. If you feel that they are making bad choices, there is nothing wrong with saying so, providing you can offer sound arguments, but do not convey the impression that their rejection of your opinion threatens your support and approval. You must work for, and desire, their independence from you.

○ WHAT TO EXPECT

The rate at which parents work through the mourning process, and acquire new knowledge and skills, varies dramatically. At one extreme are those parents who accommodate to their new situation in a few months. With such parents you may begin to feel that your intervention is redundant —that they would have managed very nicely without you.

At the other extreme are parents in whom the adjustment and learning process takes years. With such parents progress seems slow or nonexistent, and you have the impression that your efforts are wasted—that nothing will be done to meet the child's special needs until he or she is old enough to benefit from formal schooling. These parents have an uncanny knack of reminding you, from time to time, just how little progress has been made. Just when you begin to see light at the end of the tunnel, they will make some statement of belief, attitude, or hope that reminds you of the gulf between you and them and between them and their child.

Fortunately, the majority of parents falls somewhere between these extremes. They need your help, and they benefit from it. Progress is slow at times, and they may take several cycles through the mourning process, but the general feeling is that you and they are getting somewhere and that the child's needs are being met.

Much of the literature on parent guidance seems to have been written on the assumption that all hearing-impaired children are born into stable middle-class families in which the mother's main occupation is the raising of children. In fact, you may find yourself dealing with working mothers, single-parent families, cross-cultural families, bilingual homes, and parents coping with a variety of intrinsic and extrinsic problems—all of which influence the quality of the child's physical, social, and linguistic environment. To be maximally effective, you must deal with each family on its own terms. Empathy, flexibility, and creativity will be your greatest assets. If you have reached your limits and find your personal style unsuited to a particular family, do not hesitate to transfer responsibility to a colleague. You must not expect to be a success with every parent.

○ EVALUATION

Keep notes on your interactions with parents, and record particular statements or actions that reveal their progress in coming to terms with their feelings in relation to deafness and their child.

Document the topics covered in the formal educational component of your program. Remember, however, that the presentation of information is no guarantee that it has been learned. Look for, and note, any evidence that the information has been assimilated and understood.

Note the acquisition of various skills such as

1. Checking the hearing aid.
2. Drawing the child's attention to sound.
3. Using sound meaningfully.
4. Establishing dialogue with the child in activities of daily living and in play.
5. Using appropriate language.
6. Reinforcing speech skills.

Make particular note of how comfortable parents are with these activities and the extent to which they can engage in them without creating anxiety in the child.

The parental component of management represents the foundation on which the other components must rest. Through your interactions with parents you can help them explore and come to terms with their feelings; you can teach them what they need to know about deafness and its effect on child development; you can teach them the skills they need in order to facilitate their child's development; and you can help them acquire confidence in their own decision-making abilities. These goals can be accomplished during individual or group sessions. The wide variations in parent aptitudes, coping behaviors, economic situations, and social environments require teachers with knowledge, skill, empathy, flexibility, and creativity. Above all, this work requires teachers with considerable emotional integrity.

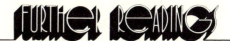

FURTHER READING

I heartily recommend David Luterman's *Counselling Parents of Hearing-Impaired Children* (Little, Brown, Boston 1979). In addition to its intrinsic merit, it is a useful source of references. You should also consult Patricia Elwood, Wayne Johnson, and Judith Mandell's *Parent-Centered Programs for Young Hearing Impaired Children* (Prince George's County Public Schools, Upper Marlboro, Md. 1977). Helmer Myklebust's *Your Deaf Child* (Chas. C Thomas, Springfield, Ill., 1950) is well worth rereading in spite of its age, and no bibliography on this topic would be complete without the *Tracy Correspondence Course for Parents* (Tracy Clinic, Los Angeles, 1964). *Parent-Infant Intervention,* edited by Audrey Simmons-Martin and Donald R. Calvert (Grune & Stratton, New York, 1979) contains several useful papers presented at an international conference.

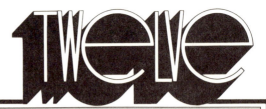

○ OBJECTIVES

○ PROCEDURES

   parent counselling

   child management

   language

   when the child enters school

○ EVALUATION

○ SUMMARY

○ FURTHER READINGS

Social and emotional management

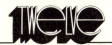

The social and emotional needs of the hearing-impaired child are the same as those of the normally hearing child. Since hearing impairment, delayed language, and negative parental reactions conspire to undermine social and emotional development, however, this topic must be given high priority in a program of management. Our concern is not only for the psychological well-being of the child. A healthy self-image and a desire for communicative interaction with other people are prerequisites for language development. For a review of this topic, please read Chapters Three and Five.

Since this issue must be handled almost exclusively through parent education and instruction, it could well have been included in the previous chapter. In order to stress its importance, however, I am treating it as a separate topic.

○ OBJECTIVES

If this aspect of management is successful, the child will:

1. Develop a healthy self-image.
2. Interact with others in age-appropriate ways.

Attainment of these goals will be demonstrated by such behaviors as

Exploration of objects and materials in the physical environment.
Exploration of the social environment through interaction and shared play.
Showing pride in achievement.
Using adults as a resource.
Seeking dialogue with adults.
Behaving differently towards different adults.
Being wary of strangers.
Expressing emotions—eventually in socially acceptable ways.
Negotiating for control and testing for limits.
Understanding and accepting the concept of ownership.
Sharing and comforting.

The only way to exert a major influence on the young child's social and emotional development is through the parents. There is little that can be done in preschool or primary school to counteract the negative effects of an unfavorable family environment.

parent counselling

The first, and most important, requirement is that the parents find their own emotional equilibrium. The longer they remain in a state of anger, denial, guilt, and confusion, the more they will reflect negative feelings back to the child. If they withhold contact and interaction, this too will work against the establishment of a good self-image and appropriate social behaviors. Those aspects of counselling that are designed to help parents come to terms with their feelings should contribute indirectly to the social and emotional well-being of the child.

child management

Beyond this, my only advice is to provide a set of guidelines. This issue must be handled with sensitivity since it carries the implication that the parents do not know how to bring up their own child. If, however, you have already discussed with them the ways in which hearing impairment undermines social and emotional development and the need to counteract this in order to provide a solid base for language development, your suggestions may be welcomed—perhaps even solicited. A possible set of guidelines follows:

1. *Demonstrate your love and affection* Provide the reassurance of physical contact. Let the child know you are happy to be with him. Follow his lead in conversation and play. Show interest in what he does. Let him see your pride and excitement in his achievements. Let him feel that he is worth spending time with. If he does something that upsets you, by all means let him know, but avoid leading him to believe that you do not like him because of what he did. Remember that the child without receptive language depends on physical contact, facial expression, intonation patterns, and gestures for positive messages about himself. In the words of Eliza Doolittle, ''Don't talk of love, show me!''

2. *Provide an interesting but safe environment for the child* It is the nature of the child to explore and to experiment or as some parents put it, ''to get into things.'' Make sure that he or she has space in which to do this by removing objects that are dangerous or valuable and by limiting access to certain places. Within the space thus defined, you should set limits (but do not expect them to be accepted promptly or permanently), and you should provide the raw materials with which the child can satisfy the need for exploration, cre-

ativity, and fantasy—toys, materials, household objects, and so on. If the child and your treasured possessions must be protected by repeated admonitions and scoldings, or if your limits are repeatedly transgressed because of boredom, the end result will be a lot of hostility and a negative self-image.

3. *Provide social variety* The only way for the child to learn about other people is to spend time with them. Include several adults and several children in his social circle, and make sure that he gets to spend time away from you. Do not expect the child under three years of age to play cooperatively with other children, and do not judge his social skills by adult standards.

4. *Strike a balance between predictability and novelty* All children need both the security of routine and the challenge of novelty, not necessarily in the same proportions. As a child develops language, he or she is able to cope with more novelty, partly because the new can be explained in terms of the old. The child without language may remain dependent on the predictable and may resist changes of routine. To the extent that it does not interfere with overall development, the need for structure can be met. At the same time, however, the child must learn to deal with new people, new places, and new experiences. As far as possible you should prepare him or her through the use of nonverbal communication—photographs, models, mementos, and so on.

5. *Set limits and apply them consistently* Make it clear to the child, and to yourself, that there are some behaviors that are required (for example, going to bed at a certain time), some behaviors that are forbidden (for example, throwing food on the floor), and some behaviors that are optional (for example, taking a teddy bear to bed). Negotiate over those things you feel flexible about but not over the others. Once you have established a social contract with the child, be consistent in its application. Whether the rules are strict or permissive is less important than that they are consistently applied. It can be very disturbing for a child to be allowed to do something one day and be punished for doing the same thing the next day. Expect the child to keep testing the limits—especially when new people are around. It is easy to interpret this behavior as naughtiness, but in fact it is a search for reassurance that things will not change. Remember that whereas the normally hearing child can test limits verbally by arguing and wheedling, the child without language must continue to test them concretely and may, therefore, give the impression of being less well behaved.

6. *Help the child learn socially acceptable ways of expressing feelings* Let the child know that you understand his or her feelings and the reasons for them. Talk about being angry, sad, disappointed, happy, and so on. Make it clear that certain behaviors, such as throwing and hitting, are unacceptable while others, such as foot stamping, are acceptable. Do not deny the child's feelings. Do not convey the impression that certain emotions should not be felt. Help the child to recognize and understand his or her feelings and to find acceptable ways of externalizing them. Remember, once again, that the child without language is at a disadvantage because of an inability to express feelings in words.

7. *Provide opportunities for creative play* Building, modelling, painting, dancing, acting, and making music are all valuable to the child. They not only provide opportunity for exploration of the physical world, but they offer a means of expressing and exploring fears, feelings, and fantasies.

8. *Be a good model* Regardless of whether the child has language or not, it is your behavior, rather than your words, that serves as a social model. You must share, empathize, comfort, express your feelings in socially acceptable ways, be creative, and take pride in your achievements. The child must see these things happen.

language

It will be seen from the foregoing that one of the keys to development of a socially and emotionally intact child is language. This is both the root of the problem and a potential solution. To a certain extent we can compensate for the absence of language by more effective use of nonverbal communication, but this does not obviate the need for early establishment of linguistic competence. It is the role of language in social and emotional development that provides one of the most cogent arguments in favor of the early use of sign language with the child for whom spoken language development is likely to be seriously delayed.

when the child enters school

Although the school environment cannot compensate for an unhealthy family environment, it can certainly reinforce a healthy one. Almost everything I have said about parent-child interactions applies equally to teacher-child interactions.

○ EVALUATION

Look for behavioral signs of a healthy self-image and age-appropriate social development. The examples given earlier in this chapter can be used as a basis for questions and comments. For example, does the child:

1. Play with objects and materials in age-appropriate ways?
2. Interact with other children and adults in age-appropriate ways?
3. Show pride in achievement?
4. Use adults as a resource?
5. Seek dialogue with adults?
6. Behave differently towards different adults?
7. Show wariness of strangers?
8. Express his or her emotions in acceptable ways?
9. Negotiate for control and test for limits?
10. Accept the concept of ownership?
11. Share with and comfort other children?

Note the use of the phrase *age appropriate*. A child's social and emotional development are intimately tied to his or her cognitive development and, therefore, follow a fairly predictable time sequence. Knowledge of this sequence is important when evaluating children or discussing their progress with parents. Showing pride in achievement, using adults as a resource, being wary of strangers, and so on are all behaviors whose emergence depends on underlying cognitive abilities. For this reason, it may be preferable to evaluate the child's social and emotional status against a standardized, norm-referenced scale.

A healthy self-image and a desire for communicative interaction with other people, apart from their intrinsic importance, are prerequisites for language development. These issues can be addressed through parent counselling in the form of guidelines for child management.

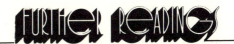

Selma Fraiberg's *The Magic Years* (Scribners, New York, 1959) has lost nothing of its freshness over the years. It includes excellent coverage of social and emotional development in normal children, as does Burton White's more recent *The First Three Years of Life* (Prentice-Hall, Inc., Englewood Cliffs, N.J., 1975). You should also read T. Gordon's *Parent Effectiveness Training* (Peter H. Wyden, Inc., New York, 1970). For in-depth treatments of the topic, I recommend Eric H. Erikson's *Childhood and Society* (W. W. Norton & Co., Inc., New York, 1963) and Eleanor Maccoby's *Social Development, Psychological Growth and the Parent-Child Relationship* (Harcourt Brace Jovanovich, Inc., New York, 1980).

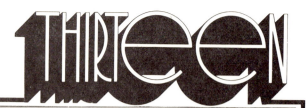

Special cases

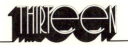

Our attention has been focussed so far on the child whose primary problem is a severe or profound sensory hearing loss and whose parents are fluent speakers of the language of his or her cultural environment. The management program I have outlined remains valid even when these conditions are not met, but certain adaptations may be necessary. These adaptations are discussed in the present chapter.

○ DEVELOPMENT AND INTERVENTION REEXAMINED

Before discussing various types of hearing impairment and possible complicating factors, it is helpful to reexamine the nature of early development and intervention.

development

In Chapter Three I described the task of the developing child as one of establishing an internal model of the world and acquiring a symbol system to provide access to that model. Between birth and age five, the child exhibits development of several functions.

1. *Sensorimotor Development* This is the first stage of development, during which children learn to attend to and associate the information generated by their sense organs in response to physical stimuli. Some of the stimuli are generated by their own movements—at first by accident and later by intent.
2. *Perceptual Development* This occurs when the child begins to interpret the physical stimuli in terms of a world of objects and events.
3. *Conceptual Development* In the next stage, the world of objects and events is reinterpreted in terms of rules, attributes, roles, relationships, causes, effects, space, and time.
4. *Social-Emotional Development* As part of conceptual development, children learn to distinguish the world of people from the world of things, and they learn that people have special rules, attributes, roles, relationships, causes, and effects. They also learn that people can be controlled by symbolic movements.
5. *Language Development* Concurrently with conceptual development children learn labels for categories within their world models; they learn rules for modifying and combining those labels to express specific ideas; they learn

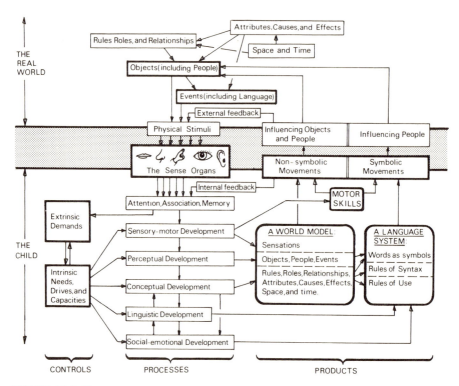

FIGURE 13–1 The process of development. In response to extrinsic demands, inner drives, and basic capacities, the child explores his environment and organizes the information provided by his senses. The result is a "world model" that represents the child's inferences about the real world. At first, this is a world of sensations and impressions. Then the sensations are interpreted in terms of objects and events. Next, the objects and events are interpreted in terms of underlying rules, roles, and relationships. Finally, the child acquires a system of symbols to represent categories within his world model. The world model can be accessed directly by sensory input (for example, seeing a cat) or indirectly via receptive language (for example, hearing the word "cat"). Similarly, the child can influence the physical world by direct movement and the social world by expressive language. Because of complex interdependencies, primary impairment of one function causes secondary impairment of other functions.

the skills necessary for generating sequences of symbolic movements and for interpreting them when expressed by others; and they learn how to influence the world of people with these movements.

These aspects of development and their associated functions are illustrated in Figure 13–1.

primary and secondary impairments

There are four prerequisites for successful progress in each area of development:

1. Intrinsic drives.

2. Basic capacities.

3. Extrinsic demands.

4. Subskills, established during earlier stages of development.

If a child lacks intrinsic drives or basic capacities, this lack constitutes a *primary impairment.* If, however, the extrinsic demands or required subskills are missing, the resulting developmental delay represents a *secondary impairment.*

It follows, from the complex nature of the developmental process, that a single, unidentified primary impairment will quickly lead to multiple secondary impairments. This phenomenon has already been discussed at length in connection with the child whose primary impairment is a malfunctioning cochlea. (See Chapters One and Five.)

roles of invervention

When developing a program of management for neurologically impaired, multiply handicapped, or environmentally disadvantaged children, it is important to consider the general goals of intervention. These include:

1. *Correction* Correction is accomplished by removing the primary impairment. In cases of conductive hearing impairments, surgical correction may be possible. In cases of conductive and sensory hearing impairment, partial prosthetic correction may be possible using hearing aids. If the primary impairment is an understimulating environment, correction may be attempted through education of parents or parent surrogates. When the primary problem is an absence of internal drives or neurologically determined capacities, the most you can hope for is some self-correction as a result of maturational processes.

2. *Delineation* An important role of early intervention is to determine the true nature of the child's difficulties. You must attempt to define and, if possible, quantify the impairments; determine which are primary and which secondary; discover which will respond to remediation; and generally describe the child's capacities, abilities, strengths, weaknesses, and optimal learning style. Evaluation of parent-child relationships and interactions is a critical component. Delineation is accomplished through observation, diagnostic teaching, and clinical assessment.

3. *Prevention* A major justification for early intervention is that it provides an opportunity for the prevention of secondary impairments. Preventive intervention is a very real possibility for children with known conductive and sensory hearing impairments. Unfortunately, many of the problems with which you must deal are not identified until secondary impairments of language development become apparent. Even if the child is in serious trouble by the time he or she comes under your influence, you may still be able to arrest the maladaptive process through effective parent counselling and education.

4. *Compensation* Sometimes it is possible to compensate for sensory or environmental deprivation at one stage of development by enrichment at another. Such is the goal of increased auditory and language stimulation for children who have recently been given hearing aids, children with a history of middle ear infections, and children from disadvantaged homes. Simple compensation will not be effective, however, when there is too much developmental asynchrony.

5. *Remediation* Remediation is an attempt to improve, or even normalize, those functions which have suffered secondary impairments. In many cases this will involve engaging the child in contrived activities that are more appropriate to an earlier stage of development (babbling, for example). In the child with a sensory hearing impairment, the goal of auditory management, subsequent to the fitting of a hearing aid, is remedial. You should note that primary impairments, as defined in this chapter, are not responsive to remedial intervention.

6. *Circumvention* When a child lacks the capacities, drives, or subskills that are normally required for progression from one stage of development to another, alternatives must be found. Examples of circumvention are the use of touch and vision for speech training with the nonauditory child and the use of sign language with the child who has not mastered speech.

○ CHILDREN WHOSE PRIMARY IMPAIRMENT IS CONDUCTIVE OR SENSORY

I have already devoted several chapters to the child with a severe or profound sensory hearing loss. This section is concerned only with children who have less severe hearing losses or hearing losses which fluctuate in severity.

mild or moderate hearing losses

A child whose primary impairment is a conductive or sensory hearing loss of less than 60 dB will develop speech and language, though imperfectly. As a result, there may be delays in identification and diagnosis which will lead to confusion on the part of the parents and add to the secondary social-emotional impairment caused by the hearing loss itself.

Corrective intervention, using hearing aids, should be very successful and with good audiological and auditory management, it should be possible to prevent further secondary handicaps. Compensation and remediation will focus on language, speech, social, and emotional issues, primarily through parent counselling and language stimulation.

You may have difficulty convincing parents and child of the necessity for full time use of the hearing aids, since aided and unaided performance will not be dramatically different. This problem must be handled through parent counselling, a clear distinction being made between the use of existing skills and the development of new ones.

Be on the lookout for signs of excessive Saturation Sound Pressure Level and excessive gain. (See Chapter Seven.) If the child resists amplification, even though these parameters have been carefully controlled, the possibility of vented earmolds should be considered. Closed earmolds exclude children's natural hearing and force them to rely on the low fidelity output of the aids. Vented molds, on the other hand, allow sound to enter the ear canal naturally and to mix with the output of the aid. If venting causes feedback problems, a CROS fitting may be necessary, in which the child wears the microphone over one ear and the rest of the aid over the other. It is imperative that the parents understand the rationale for such things as venting and CROS fitting and that they monitor the aids scrupulously. Since aided and unaided performance are very similar, it will be easy for faults to go undetected.

When the time comes for enrollment in a nursery program, the obvious choice will be for full mainstreaming. Placement decisions should, however, take account of the acoustic environment. The child with a mild or moderate hearing loss will have great difficulty coping with high noise levels, reverberant rooms, and large class sizes. Once he or she is enrolled, a program of in-service orientation must be provided for the child's teachers.

unilateral hearing losses

Loss of hearing in one ear, even though it represents a 50 percent reduction of auditory input, does not appear to cause serious developmental problems. The otherwise intact child adapts to this condition, and in the days before mandatory screening, it was not uncommon for total unilateral hearing losses to go undetected until adulthood. This does not mean that there are no consequences, however. Sound localization and speech perception in noise are both affected, and the child has particular trouble in a noisy environment when the speaker is on his "bad" side. If the loss is discovered in early childhood, it is important that parents and preschool teachers be made aware of its implications and that a program of hearing conservation be instituted. I do not, however, recommend amplification for children with severe or profound unilateral losses, since any acoustic benefits are usually offset by cosmetic and maintenance problems.

Children with a mild or moderate hearing loss in one ear are, ironically, in more jeopardy than are children with a severe or profound unilateral loss. This is because they receive different neural messages from the two cochleas —one of which only functions when sounds are moderately loud. This confusion may lead to problems of auditory attention and difficulties with speech perception. Although I have no research data to support this, it has been my clinical impression that moderate unilateral losses are more serious when they are on the right side. This would certainly be anticipated since the right cochlea makes more neurological connections with the left cerebral hemisphere than it does with the right, and since the left hemisphere is dominant for language.

I do recommend amplification for children with a mild or moderate unilateral hearing loss so that they may receive consistent auditory input from both cochleas. I also recommend formal, but low level, intervention with the primary emphasis on auditory attention and speech perception.

fluctuating hearing losses

Perceptual development requires reliable sense organs. Only with a consistent and predictable relationship between physical stimuli and neural messages can the developing child learn to interpret the information received from the environment. Periodic fluctuations of sensitivity cause confusion, with a consequent lowering of priority for the modality concerned.

Such is the situation of the young child with recurring ear infections. Until the mid-1970s these infections were thought to be a purely medical problem with negligible effects on development. It is now realized that the child whose hearing sensitivity fluctuates may well develop secondary auditory perceptual problems, possibly leading to learning disabilities.

The main difficulty seems to be one of auditory attention. The children stop listening, because their ears are unreliable. Unless remedied, this problem leads to delays of speech and language development. Some authorities recommend both prosthetic and habilitative intervention for all children who experience six or more ear infections in the first two years of life. A low power hearing aid is fitted monaurally and its use continued even during periods of normal hearing. The purpose of the aid is to provide consistency of auditory stimulation. Habilitative intervention is limited to parent education and instruction with a view to enriching the child's experience of spoken language, thus preventing secondary impairments.

○ CHILDREN WHOSE PRIMARY IMPAIRMENT IS NEURAL

In this section I discuss children with impairments of the neural mechanism of hearing as well as those whose auditory behavior is abnormal because of other kinds of neurological damage.

auditory processing disorders

Children with auditory processing disorders have problems with the interpretation of sound patterns, even when their sensitivity and discrimination capacity are adequate for the task at hand. Such difficulties manifest themselves in several ways. For example,

1. Sounds do not attract the child's attention.
2. The child cannot attend to an auditory message when there is competition from visual or tactile messages or inner thoughts.
3. The child cannot attend to one auditory message when there is competition from another auditory message (even though the latter is not loud enough to cause real masking).
4. The child cannot remember the first part of a sound pattern while waiting for a later part.
5. The child does not learn to associate sound patterns with the objects and events which cause them (and, therefore, does not learn to recognize sounds).
6. Individual sound patterns in a sequence are recognized, but their order is forgotten.
7. The child cannot use the auditory channel for activities involving comprehension or symbolic function.

Some of these behaviors are easily confused with the effects of sensory hearing impairment—even in the clinic. Misdiagnosis is therefore a strong possibility, especially in young children.

When auditory processing disorders are secondary to the effects of delayed amplification, fluctuating hearing loss, or excessive environmental noise, they may be reversible. As primary impairments, however, they are irreversible, although there may be some spontaneous recovery in the child whose neural mechanism has been damaged by such things as anoxia or bacteria.

You should note that the term *auditory processing disorder* is very general and probably includes a variety of conditions. It is possible, for example, that many auditory problems are essentially temporal disorders in which the child has difficulty perceiving simultaneity and sequence or making decisions in the time available. Such problems manifest themselves in auditory tasks for the simple reason that sounds are basically patterns in time. The child with temporal difficulties should not have trouble with the auditory perception of space, but he or she will have difficulty with visual-temporal tasks such as lipreading and the reading of fingerspelling.

Mild disorders of auditory processing will probably go undetected until the child starts having problems in school. Severe disorders, however, will cause delays of speech and language development, and it is in this guise that they will come to your attention during the preschool years.

Most of the research on this topic has been concerned with establishing a relationship between learning disabilities and auditory problems. Remedial programs have been written and implemented with school age children, but there is little concrete evidence to show either that auditory perception improves with training or that such improvements alleviate the learning disability. The literature on auditory processing disorders in children below age five is very sparse.

Chapters Seven and Eight on audiological and auditory management may be taken as a starting point for intervention but with a major focus on delineation through diagnostic teaching. If the child has difficulty with a specific auditory task, you should investigate his ability to perform an analogous task through the visual or tactile modalities.

To compensate for some of the child's underlying problems, you can try working in a distraction free environment. You may also find it helpful to give the child extra time to reach auditory perceptual decisions. If the auditory problems are severe and irreversible, the child's linguistic and communicative needs must be met by circumventing the auditory modality and using the tactile or visual modalities.

other neurological disorders

It is quite possible that you will become responsible, either by default or design, for children with a wide variety of neurologically determined developmental disorders. Presumably there will be some question about the existence of a primary hearing impairment. The disorders may be of general perceptual organization, conceptual organization, social-emotional function, symbolic function, or language function, either separately or in combination. The children may be described by such labels as mulitply handicapped, neurologically impaired, mentally retarded, autistic, behaviorally disturbed, and aphasic.

To the extent that you accept responsibility for management, your priorities should be

1. *Delineation* Determine whether there is a primary conductive or sensory hearing impairment, and arrange for appropriate corrective intervention.

   Through diagnostic teaching, observation, and formal evaluation attempt to define the child's status within a developmental scheme such as that described earlier in this chapter. Find out also whether the symbolic and language difficulties are restricted to the motor acoustic symbols of speech.

2. *Prevention and Compensation* Through parent counselling, as well as your own interactions with the child, try to adapt the environment so as to meet immediate developmental needs and prevent the appearance of further secondary impairments. This may also give the child time to benefit from the effects of maturation.

If it becomes clear that the child's major problems are not due to a hearing impairment, you should take steps to transfer management responsibility to someone who is qualified to deal with developmentally disordered children. Even before then you should insist on the involvement of other professionals with expertise in the management of the various disabilities exhibited by the child.

mutiply handicapped children

In a sense, all of the children discussed in this book are multiply handicapped since they have secondary impairments in addition to a primary impairment. I think, however, that the term should be reserved for children who have two or more primary handicaps.

The consequences of a primary impairment of the conductive or sensory hearing mechanism tend to be magnified when there are additional primary impairments. This effect is especially marked when the other impairments are of the type just discussed, but it also occurs with impairments of sensory and motor function. A severe sensory hearing loss presents greater difficulties of management when it coexists with blindness or cerebral palsy.

Once again, you may take the outline presented in earlier chapters as a starting point for a program of management but with major emphasis on delineation and a readiness to adapt your procedures to compensate for the additional primary impairment(s).

behavior modification

The principles of reinforcement and extinction by operant conditioning can be applied to the management of hearing-impaired and multiply handicapped children—in fact, they underlie much of what I have said about development and intervention. It is wrong, however, to apply behavior modification techniques indiscriminately. Before you attempt to extinguish a particular behavior you must ask why it exists. Sometimes a behavior which seems infantile and inappropriate may represent a very genuine and useful adaptation to the impairment on the part of the child. Consider, for example, the child with severe neurologically determined delays of development who, at three and a half years of age still puts everything in his mouth. To extinguish this behavior because it seems inappropriate may be to deprive the child of his one effective channel for exploration and sensorimotor development. Unfortunately, it is easier to focus on observable behavior than to delineate a complex network of underlying causes. If you do attempt to extinguish behaviors, you must determine what needs they are meeting and find alternative ways of meeting those needs.

○ ENVIRONMENTAL COMPLICATIONS

Children develop not only according to internal processes but also by interactions with their physical and social environment. The environment provides a stimulus for development, reinforcement of behaviors, and a forum for the rehearsal and refinement of perceptual, motor, conceptual, social, and linguistic skills. I have already discussed how instinctive parental reactions serve to complicate the development of the hearing-impaired child. In a sense these reactions may be thought of as a secondary impairment. But what happens if there is a primary impairment in the physical and social environment? Examples of such impairment might be the absence of play materials, the withholding of human interaction, or constraints on language input because of the parents' own language difficulties.

environmental deprivation

An otherwise intact child who grows in an impoverished environment will exhibit mild or moderate secondary impairments in many areas of development, including auditory perception. Unfortunately, the parents who create this environment will probably not seek professional help during the preschool years. The situation you are most likely to encounter is one in which an impoverished home environment is a complication of a severe or profound sensory hearing loss. In such cases, the prognosis is poor. It is unlikely that your best efforts at parent counselling will produce dramatic changes in attitudes or behaviors, and it is the parents who are the key to intervention. Compensatory intervention will therefore be high on your list of priorities. You must involve the child in one-to-one or group learning situations for as much of the day as possible and as early as possible.

Cultural factors play an important role in determining the quality of a child's social and physical environment. If the parents grew up in a society which views childhood merely as a temporary and somewhat inconvenient stage on the way to adulthood, they may have difficulty adapting to the special needs of a hearing-impaired child. You may have success with parent counselling if the parents are reasonably intelligent and genuinely concerned, but once again you must give high priority to compensatory intervention in a clinical or nursery school setting.

It has been suggested that environmental and social understimulation can be the sole cause of severe impairments of social-emotional function—manifesting themselves as autistic behavior. I find it difficult to believe that the neurologically intact child would respond in this way unless grossly maltreated. If, however, an understimulating environment interacts with primary neurological impairments, such an outcome is more explicable.

bilingual parents

The normally hearing, neurologically intact child has little difficulty acquiring two or more languages simultaneously. The child with a hearing impairment, however, has difficulty learning one language and more difficulty still if exposed to a second language. It follows that bilingual parents should decide which language their child will learn and avoid exposing him or her to others.

For truly bilingual parents, that is, parents who are equally fluent in both languages, the choice is obvious. They should allow their child to acquire the language of their new social environment, even though this may not be their native language.

Unfortunately, most situations that are described as bilingual are really monolingual with a smattering of a second language. This creates a serious dilemma. If the parents decide that their child's first language shall be their own native language, he may need to learn a second language in school. If, on the other hand, they decide to use the language of their adopted country, they will provide poor models, they will create an artifical barrier between themselves and their child, and they will most probably isolate him from general family conversations. A complicating factor with many immigrant families is that the father acquires fluency because of his work and he decides that the mother must use the new language. The mother, in the meantime, has minimal contact with native speakers of the new language and, therefore, has little opportunity to acquire fluency. There is a good chance that she will resent being given this additional burden, especially when she has been uprooted from her native culture and the support of her family.

Having watched several families struggle with this problem, I am of the opinion that the child should acquire the native language of his or her parents unless it is clear that they are *both* committed to acquiring mastery of the new language. This presupposes, of course, that you or a colleague are also fluent in the parents' language. This approach still places an educational burden on the child when he or she enters school, but I believe that the social and emotional integrity of the child and family must be given top priority.

The foregoing comments also apply to the early use of sign language by normally hearing parents. This option only makes sense when the parents are fully committed to the acquisition of fluency in this new language modality—to the extent that they are prepared to use it for all family interactions in which the child is a potential participant. In the absence of such a commitment, the child will receive poor models, he or she will be communicatively isolated from the rest of the family, and the quality of the relationship between child and parents will suffer.

hearing-impaired parents

When the parents of a hearing-impaired child are themselves hearing-impaired, they do not usually go through the mourning process discussed in Chapter Five. Consequently, they are able to provide a warm, stimulating, and communicatively effective environment without your help. They will, however, have problems meeting the child's needs for audiological, auditory, and speech management. There are two ways to deal with this. One is to include normally hearing family members in the habilitative process and let them serve as surrogate parents for the hearing and speech components. The other is to provide compensatory intervention either in the clinic or by early enrollment in a nursery program.

The same approach should be used with normally hearing children of hearing-impaired parents. They must be given every opportunity to hear normal speech and to interact with normally hearing relatives, surrogate parents, clinicians, or teachers. These comments apply to both oral deaf parents and manual deaf parents.

The young child's progress is influenced by extrinsic demands, inner drives, basic capacities, and the existence of subskills established during earlier stages of development. Because of this interdependence of intrinsic and extrinsic factors, a primary impairment of one function can produce secondary impairments of other functions. Intervention is aimed at correction of the primary impairment, delineation of all impairments, prevention of secondary impairments, compensation for sensory or environmental deprivation, remediation of secondary impairments, and circumvention. Priorities depend on the nature of the child's difficulties and circumstances. For mild, moderate, and unilateral hearing losses, correction and prevention are the main goals. For fluctuating hearing losses, correction, prevention, and remediation may be necessary. Auditory processing disorders, other neurological disorders, and multiple handicaps call for delineation, compensation, remediation, and possible circumvention. Complications such as environmental, social, and linguistic deprivation may be viewed as primary impairments. They are potentially correctible but will most probably require compensatory intervention with the child.

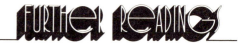

The topic of mild fluctuating hearing losses is dealt with in Burton Jaffe's *Hearing Loss in Children* (University Park Press, Baltimore, Md., 1977) and Jerry Northern and Marion Downs' *Hearing in Children—second edition* (Williams & Wilkins, Baltimore, Md., 1978).

For information on the diagnosis of auditory processing and other neurologically determined communication disorders, I refer you to Helmer Myklebust's *Auditory Disorders in Children* (Grune & Stratton, New York, 1954) which is still extremely useful despite advances in terminology; Patricia Cole and Mary Wood's chapter on "Differential Diagnosis" in *Pediatric Audiology* edited by F. N. Martin (Prentice Hall, Inc., Englewood Cliffs, N.J., 1978); and the chapter on "Clinical Audiological Testing" in *Hearing in Children.* (See previous paragraph.) Ian Taylor's book on *Neurological Mechanisms of Hearing and Speech in Children* (Manchester University Press, Manchester, U.K., 1964) is also worth reading. The topic of management at the preschool level is not well covered in the literature. Recommendations for differential diagnosis and diagnostic teaching are about as much as most writers have to offer.

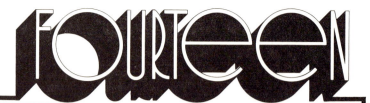

FOURTEEN

Delivery

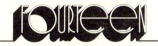

The final chapter is concerned with the logistics of early habilitative intervention and the preparation of personnel to carry out this work.

○ PARENT-INFANT WORK

The hearing-impaired child's parents are virtually your sole avenue for intervention while he or she is under three years of age. They must acquire the skills involved in day-to-day management of audiological, auditory, cognitive, linguistic, social, emotional, and communicative needs. If they are to do this effectively, they must come to terms with their own feelings, and they must learn about such things as hearing impairment, language, and child development. (See Chapter Eleven.)

There are several possible formats for a program of parent-infant management. For example

1. Schedule weekly, or biweekly, meetings during which you show the parents what to do, observe them, and offer constructive criticism. Counselling and education can occur simultaneously and incidentally, though it is probably advisable to have some sessions that are exclusively devoted to these issues. The parent guidance sessions can last anywhere from one to two hours, and they can take place either in the child's home or in the school, or center, or clinic with which you are affiliated. If the latter site is chosen, it may be helpful to create a model home, or apartment, in which you can demonstrate such things as bathing the baby, preparing food, making the bed, and so on.

2. As an alternative, or addition, to periodic individual sessions, it can be helpful to organize intensive group programs lasting for several days. Geographic and logistical constraints may make this option attractive for certain parents, and it permits efficient use of resources. By bringing several families together, you will provide a balance between individual and group sessions and also between instruction, education, and counselling. Outside specialists can be called in to enrich and extend such a program.

3. Yet another possibility is the correspondence course. This format was made famous by the John Tracy Clinic. It met the needs of countless families around the world at a time when early intervention programs barely existed at a local level. By assigning each family to a specific staff member and establishing two-way communication, it is possible to address individual needs and circumstances and to remove some of the impersonality associated with a formal written curriculum.

Whatever format you choose for this aspect of management, you must evaluate its effectiveness in terms of success in meeting the needs of the parents and achieving the goals of intervention.

○ INDIVIDUAL WORK

While the child is below three years of age, the time you spend with him or her will be devoted mainly to demonstration and diagnostic teaching. There is, however, one aspect of development for which you need to take responsibility—the initial development of speech sounds. (See Chapter Ten.)

After the child reaches two and a half or three years of age, he or she can benefit directly from one-to-one interaction with a teacher. The major focus will be language and communication skills, but within the context of the child's cognitive and social function.

I believe these sessions should last between 20 and 40 minutes, depending on the age of the child and the frequency with which he or she is seen. Ideally, there will be five sessions a week.

Even when much of the child's learning is taking place in one-to-one instruction, it is imperative that the parent management program continue. The parents must be kept fully informed of the goals of training and the progress of the child, and they must be shown how to sustain and reinforce new skills.

○ PRESCHOOL

At around three years of age, the child will be ready for a preschool experience. This will provide a stimulus for cognitive and social development and should sustain and reinforce the growth of communication skills. Preschool should also provide the child with certain readiness skills in anticipation of kindergarten.

There are several choices of format for this aspect of delivery. For example

1. *Mainstreaming* The hearing-impaired child may be enrolled in a program for normally hearing children but with three provisos:

   Additional time must be provided for both one-to-one teaching and parent guidance.

   The staff of the preschool must be given education, guidance, and support.

   The child's language skills must be sufficiently well developed to permit meaningful verbal interaction with peers and teachers.

2. *Self-contained classes* There are several advantages to teaching hearing-impaired preschoolers in a small group. This arrangement uses teaching staff efficiently and makes it possible for language and communication needs to be addressed almost exclusively. Some of the drawbacks of this traditional model are as follows:

> The auditory capacities and individual special needs of the children are likely to vary considerably and, therefore, be difficult to address in group activities.

> There is a danger of focusing on language-related needs to the exclusion of underlying cognitive, social, and emotional needs. It is very easy for parents and teachers to lose their frames of reference if their attention is focussed entirely on hearing-impaired children.

3. *Reverse mainstreaming* A compromise possibility is reverse mainstreaming. This involves adding normally hearing children to a group of hearing-impaired children. The advantages of this arrangement include:

> The appointment of full time, specialist staff is justified, and their time can be used efficiently.

> The normally hearing children provide developmental models for the hearing-impaired children, the staff, and the parents.

> The parents of hearing-impaired children can benefit from mutual support, while their interactions with the parents of normally hearing children provide a realistic frame of reference.

The disadvantages include:

> It is not the most cost-effective arrangement.

> The staff must include one or more specialists in early childhood education.

> Considerable expertise and planning are necessary if there is to be true interaction between the hearing and the hearing-impaired children.

> This kind of program mainly addresses the social, cognitive, and readiness needs of the hearing-impaired child. It must be supplemented by individual work on language and communication and by parent guidance.

Some teachers express concern that in reverse mainstreaming, normally hearing students might learn inappropriate behaviors from the hearing-impaired students. In my experience this is not a problem. Some imitation does occur, but unless reinforced, it is soon abandoned in favor of more rewarding behaviors.

If you are contemplating the establishment of a reverse mainstreaming program, or of adding normally hearing children to an existing program, you should:

> Aim for a majority of normally hearing children.

> Plan at least 20 minutes a day of individual work for the hearing-impaired children.

> Train teachers and assistants to avoid the natural tendency to spend most of their time interacting with the normally hearing children. (You will find that the

language skills of a normally hearing preschooler are a powerful means of seizing and holding the attention of adults.)

Decide how the program will be structured in order to encourage interaction between hearing and hearing-impaired children and to make such interaction successful and rewarding.

Expect some reluctance from parents of normally hearing children in the beginning. Once you have set up a first-class preschool program that provides a good learning experience for any child, regardless of hearing status, your program will sell itself. At first, however, you may have to think of ways of recruiting normally hearing students.

Screen your normally hearing applicants. One normally hearing child with behavioral problems can seriously sap the time and energy of staff and direct efforts away from the hearing-impaired children.

Within each of these three formats there are various organizational possibilities. The program can be structured or unstructured; the activities can be student-directed or teacher-directed; the emphasis can be on cooperation or on independence; the focus can be on problem solving, on creativity, or on readiness skills, and so on. Numerous texts have been written on the purpose and design of preschool programs for normally hearing children, and numerous philosophies have been put into practice. It is a characteristic of intact children from healthy and supportive home environments that they grow and learn in any educational setting, regardless of its inherent strengths and weaknesses. Hearing-impaired children are not intact, however, and it is possible that certain program formats will be incompatible with their special problems and needs. As you evaluate the suitability of a particular program for a particular child, you should ask the following questions:

1. Is the environment reasonably quiet and conducive to good hearing aid use and effective auditory development?

2. Is there sufficient predictability to compensate for the child's language deficit?

3. Is there sufficient variety to stimulate cognitive and linguistic development?

4. Does the program address the child's needs in terms of cognitive and thinking skills

   AND creativity and self-expression, AND orientation to reading and math, AND social and emotional development, AND language and communication?

5. Does the staff understand the linguistic, communicative, and social implications of hearing impairment?

6. Has provision been made for the child's special needs in relation to audiological, auditory, linguistic, and communicative management?

Before leaving the topic of preschool, I must make one last comment. There is a tendency to think that once a child enters school, the parent guidance phase of management is finished. In fact, the child's parents will continue to be the primary influence on growth and development for many years. Parent education and counselling should continue through the pre-school years, regardless of program format. There is, indeed, no stage in the education of a hearing-impaired child when this component of management becomes unnecessary.

○ BEING THERE

This section is included for the benefit of the inexperienced teacher. All too often, such teachers have passed through training programs that touch only superficially on the various topics discussed in this book and in which the opportunities for supervised practicum are severely limited. To make matters worse, many find themselves working independently, with little or no access to supervision, guidance, or in-service training.

My purpose in this section is to bring a sense of synthesis and realism to a discussion that so far has been biased towards analysis and abstraction. Imagine, if you will, that you have just been given responsibility for the habilitative management of a little boy with a severe or profound hearing loss.

before you begin

Before your first encounter with the child and his family, prepare yourself by reading all relevant reports and correspondence. Look for factual details concerning pre- and perinatal history; developmental milestones; medical history; educational history; results of audiological, neurological, and psychological evaluations; and so on. Be on your guard, however, about remarks by clinicians and teachers, such as "lack of cooperation" or "manipulative parents." These comments sometimes tell you more about the clinicians than they do about their clients. Your purpose should be to develop your own mental image of the child and his family without being prejudiced by the reactions and opinions of other professionals. At the same time you should note data that may become significant as you develop a program of intervention. If other professionals are to be involved in the child's management (for example, an otologist, audiologist, or social worker), you should talk to them about the case—not so much to gain information as to open up channels of communication and support.

first encounters

Your first few meetings with the child should have two main goals —observation and the establishment of rapport. Do not feel compelled to

begin language work immediately. Get to know the child, and more importantly, give him time to get to know and trust you. Offer physical contact but
do not force it upon him. Remember that the child who's world you are
invading needs time both to assimilate and to accommodate.

Do not expect this little boy to sit with you and work at a desk. Follow
him to his territory—the floor. Remember also that young children are gross
motor rather than fine motor creatures. Be prepared to move around. It will
eventually be your responsibility to make the child feel comfortable in more
structured environments, but remember that one of the keys to dialogue is
shared control. Show the child that you will meet him half way.

When it is time to be directive, act with confidence. Nothing destroys the
trust of children and parents more than signs of hesitation or uncertainty.
This does not mean that you must be infallible and inflexible. Confidence
is not shown by having an answer for everything and never backing down.
The truly confident person is the one who can, when necessary, say, "I don't
know," "I made a mistake," or "That was a bad idea, and we are going to
try something else." Note, also, that as you attempt to direct the child, you
should move in small steps. Try to avoid backing yourself into a corner from
which the only escape is a battle of wills.

It is possible that the child will, at first, refuse to interact with you,
clinging instead to his mother.* Be patient and take your time. Unless there
are serious problems in the mother-child relationship, the nervous child will
eventually come around. Play by yourself for a while, occasionally acknowledging his presence, offering participation, or leaving some part of your play
material where it can be reached without the child having to stray too close
to you or too far from his mother. Sometimes you can speed things up by
leaving the room for five or ten minutes. Some children need a chance to
explore a new environment in mother's presence before they feel secure
enough to take on the additional challenge of a new person. When you
return, it is as though you were coming into his territory instead of inviting
him into yours. If you are still unsuccessful, do not worry. There will be
more sessions. Above all, reassure the parents that this behavior is not
unusual and that you are not concerned about it. You will gain nothing by
exacerbating the mother's feelings of guilt or inadequacy.

Whether or not the child interacts directly with you, you should observe
him. Note, for example, his approach to new objects and to new people, his
general level of activity, and his ability to stay on topic. Ask whether his
activity is focussed or random. Note how he deals with problems. Does he
attack them without apparent plan? Does he give up easily? Does he perse-
verate in an attempted solution in spite of repeated failure? Does he try
alternative solutions? Does he automatically turn to his mother for help

---

*I am using the word *mother* here to refer to the person with whom the child has
established his primary interpersonal bond. This person is usually the biological
mother, but may be the father or other caregiver.

and/or approval? Does he seek your assistance and/or approval? Observe his prelanguage behavior. Does he respond to sounds, especially those of the human voice? Does he initiate dialogue? Does he insist on getting his message across? Does he seek information from speech? Does he try to use speech? There is little you can do with this information immediately, but it will help you form a more complete image of the child and may be useful in planning an overall intervention program or in understanding why specific approaches are not working.

Although your main concerns are observation and rapport, you should come to these early sessions well prepared. Select "topics" that you think may be suitable for your dialogue—either toys, daily living activities, or both. Take into account the child's age and developmental level, and remember the limited attention span of small children. It is better to have too much material than too little. Do not let it be obvious, however, that you are drawing from a pool of toys, or the child may try to work through them all as quickly as possible. Be alert for early signs of boredom so that you can take the initiative in changing topic. Above all, be flexible. At least 50 percent of your dialogue should be directed by the child's immediate interests (for example, his bruised knee, your watch) or by the unexpected (for example, a squirrel on the window ledge).

Your early sessions with the parents should similarly be used for observation and the establishment of rapport. Do not overwhelm them with interrogation, factual information, or instruction. Take the time to talk with them —listening to their stories, their concerns, and their feelings. Observe how they interact with their child. Look for signs of anxiety. Note whether they are using you as a resource to help them solve their own problems or whether they expect you to take the problems from them. Note differences of behavior when the parents are seen together or separately. Ask whether the parents agree with each other on the subject of their child and his management.

A primary goal in your early meetings with the parents should be to reduce the level of any anxiety that is present. Reassure them that the most important things they can do for their child are to play with him, to talk to him, and to enjoy him. If you are dealing with a situation in which, because of other demands, neither parent can spend a lot of time with the child, try to reassure them that quality of interaction is more important than quantity, but look into the possibility of including in your program the person (or persons) who *will* be taking care of him. Remember that any short term gains you make by playing on the parents' guilt in order to meet the child's communicative needs may generate hidden hostilities that serve only to undermine the social-emotional foundations of his long term development.

There are, unfortunately, increasing numbers of parents who do not enjoy their children—with or without a hearing impairment. The causes can be several: Possibly their own childhoods were not very enjoyable; perhaps they grew up in a culture that regards childhood as a temporary inconvenience; or perhaps their needs to raise and nurture children are in conflict with other needs, such as financial solvency, greater affluence, professional advancement, or a search for identity. A former colleague, Dr. Angela Broomfield, expressed the problem concisely when, after an exhausting day of parent guidance, she said, "I spend so much of my time trying to teach parents how to play with their children!" Unfortunately, this is not a situation in which teaching can be very effective. Perhaps, with long term counselling, you can help such parents to greater self-understanding and an internally motivated reordering of priorities, but in most cases the prognosis is not good. Once again, be patient and avoid the temptation to play on the parents' guilt in order to pressure them into doing what you think is good for the child.

Soon after your program of intervention begins, you should visit the child in his home. Such a visit is advisable regardless of the eventual location of your meetings. It will give you a more complete understanding of the child and his family and should help them develop the trust that is so important to the success of your work.

Another contributor to parental trust will be your openness. Share with them your goals for these early sessions, and give them a rough outline of the changes you will make once everyone feels comfortable together. Anything you do to develop trust in the parents should also help develop trust in the child. Children have no difficulty determining when their parents are angry or happy, anxious or comfortable, afraid or confident, suspicious or trusting, and so on and are always ready to adopt these reactions.

Although I have stressed the need to postpone your assault on the child's communicative needs, there is one practical issue that must be addressed from the outset—hearing aid monitoring. You should begin every session by examining and listening to the hearing aids yourself, and as soon as possible, the parents should be checking the aids once or twice a day. Set time aside for instruction in hearing aid monitoring, and arrange for someone else to take the child for a few minutes while you do this so that the parents will not be distracted. Keep two or three defective aids around to demonstrate what the parents should listen for, and show them how to test the batteries.

later sessions

Once you have developed a knowledge of your clients and established a comfortable working relationship in which there is play dialogue with the child and verbal dialogue with his parents, you should be ready to address their more obvious needs—cognition, language, speech, and hearing for the child; grieving, knowledge, skills, and independence for his parents.

As you play with the child, introduce moments that require him to do one or more of the following:

1. Solve problems.	(See Chapter Nine.)
2. Attend to sound patterns.	(See Chapter Eight.)
3. Interpret sound patterns.	(See Chapter Eight.)
4. Attend to language patterns.	(See Chapter Nine.)
5. Interpret language patterns.	(See Chapter Nine.)
6. Imitate speech movements.	(See Chapter Ten.)
7. Use speech to express language.	(See Chapters Nine and Ten.)

Sometimes, when introducing a new activity, or a new twist to an old activity, you may need to spend a large part of a session on one item from the previous list. For the most part, however, these items should be interwoven into your dialogue. Each session should be fun, and its purpose, from the child's perspective, should be unrelated to teaching. Your task is to maintain an enjoyable and purposeful dialogue, whose form requires the child to engage in behaviors that promote a synthesis of social, emotional, auditory, cognitive, and communicative development.

As with first encounters, you should begin each session by checking the hearing aids, and you should come well prepared. Preparation requires not only a decision about materials and activities but also a set of goals related to the various aspects of development with which you are concerned. You must have in your mind a series of stages through which you expect the child to progress, one such series for each developmental area, an assessment of the child's present status in each area, and a clear idea of where you want him to go next. I am not suggesting an inflexible game plan with specific behavioral objectives at each level. You must always be prepared to change your ideas as their inadequacies are illuminated by real children and your own experience. Nevertheless, you must have an overall plan, an assessment of the current status, and several immediate goals.

Although your ultimate goal for parents is that they too will interact with their child in ways that facilitate development in all areas simultaneously, do not expect this kind of synthesis immediately. Until they have acquired the necessary knowledge, confidence, and skills, you will need to focus their attention on specific aspects of interaction during demonstration and instruction. At first, for example, the main focus should be on dialogue through play, with emphasis on topics, turn taking, and shared control. Then you should introduce the idea of language as an accompaniment to play dialogue, with emphasis on the need for language that parallels the messages being exchanged, the need for repetition, and the need to provide the language for the child as well as themselves. Attention can then be drawn to the possible ways to promote listening, language recognition, and language expression during interaction. At various times you may need to focus on social-emotional issues, choice of play materials, proper use of hearing aids, and so on. What I am suggesting is that you try to avoid overwhelming the parents by dealing with too many issues at once. Let them progress in small steps, dealing with one issue at a time, slowly developing an interactive style that is both helpful to the child and second nature to them. Only in this way can you hope to build the self-confidence that is the key to the parents' eventual independence from you.

The exact choice of issues, the order in which they are presented, the length of time you dwell on each one, and the number of times you return to each one must, of course, be determined by the parents' needs and rate of progress. As you observe them interact with their child, ask about the quality of that interaction in terms of social, emotional, auditory, cognitive, and communicative development. Note the areas in which you see an immediate potential for improvement, and select one as a topic for discussion and demonstration. Choose a goal that is attainable within the time available (for example, avoidance of pronouns for objects whose names are not yet in the child's vocabulary). There will be plenty of time to return to other issues later.

Avoid conveying to parents the message, "You are doing things in the wrong way, and I am going to show you the right way." Rather let them hear, "What you are doing is good, but I'm going to suggest a way of making it better." To this end, you should point out the good features of the parents' interactive style as often as you draw attention to features that need improvement. Once again, remember that your goal is to build self-confidence —not to destroy it.

○ PERSONNEL

There is no single discipline that provides complete preparation for persons undertaking early habilitative intervention. To do justice to this work you must acquire knowledge and skills from such fields as audiology, speech and language pathology, psycholinguistics, developmental psychology, counselling, social work, early childhood education, and education of the deaf.

There is an unfortunate tendency for persons trained in only one of these disciplines to assume full responsibility for management in the mistaken belief that they know all that needs to be known about the subject. Audiologists, for example, may argue that early habilitative intervention is their job because it involves hearing impairments and hearing aids; speech pathologists may claim the role because speech and language problems are the most visible symptoms of hearing impairment; but if parental reactions and family dynamics are the key to success, perhaps the psychologist or social worker has a prior claim. "No," says the teacher of the deaf, "The problem is deafness, and that is my area of expertise."

In fact, as preparation for a career in early intervention, the basic training of all these professionals is uniformly incomplete. Each holds some pieces to the jigsaw, but none has the complete puzzle.

When a particular task requires skills and knowledge from a variety of disciplines, there are two options: Organize a team in which each discipline is represented, or take a person from one of the disciplines and provide him or her with additional training in the others.

Much has been written about the team approach to early intervention, and in theory it provides the best of everything. Unfortunately, a team is more than an assembly of professionals. It requires structure, communication, coordination, and leadership if it is to function effectively. On more than one occasion I have watched constructive discussions about the merits of the team approach degenerate into arguments about who should be in charge. Another problem with the team approach is that it virtually presupposes a large, accessible population of children to be served, a condition that applies only in urban centers. Given such a population and good organization and leadership, the team approach undoubtedly has much to offer.

In practice, however, early habilitative intervention has been undertaken most frequently and most effectively by individuals who have travelled beyond the boundaries of their own disciplines in order to acquire additional skills and knowledge. In such cases the most significant factors have been ability and determination, rather than primary qualification. A *Who's Who* of leaders in this field would show them to come from numerous disciplines, including education, psychology, audiology, speech pathology, medicine, and even dentistry. In the 1970s, there evolved a few training programs in North America with the specific goal of preparing personnel to work in this field. Even if you have been enrolled in one of these programs (and especially if you have not), you must continue to increase your expertise by reading, coursework, observation, and supervised practicum. If your situation requires you to take primary responsibility for management, you should establish a support system that allows you to call on professionals from other disciplines when you have reached the limits of your own knowledge or skill.

Intervention with the very young child must occur within the framework of parental guidance. As the child matures, he or she will benefit from a mixture of individual communication therapy and enrollment in a preschool. The preschool experience may be self-contained, or it may involve various levels of mainstreaming.

When working with a new child, inform yourself about his or her status and history, and use the first few sessions to observe and to establish rapport. Your goal must be to establish a comfortable play dialogue. You may then introduce activities that put pressure on the development of cognitive, auditory, linguistic, and speech skills. Your goal is to maintain a synthesis in which all developmental areas are addressed in synchrony and in ways that permit one area to influence or be influenced by others. At the same time, the child must perceive more immediate and more concrete goals that will maintain his or her interest, enthusiasm, and cooperation.

A similar progression should be followed with the parents, except that synthesis can be delayed to give them time to assimilate knowledge and acquire skills in specific areas. Your interactions with parents should foster self-confidence.

No traditional discipline prepares professionals fully for early habilitative intervention with hearing-impaired children. Successful programs require either a team approach or the willingness of individuals to acquire knowledge and skills that go beyond their basic training.

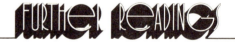

David Luterman's *Counselling Parents of Hearing-Impaired Children* (Little Brown, Boston, 1979) contains a review of program options for the parent aspect of this work. Another useful source, to which I have already made extensive reference, is Patricia Elwood, Wayne Johnson, and Judith Mandell's *Parent-Centered Programs for Young Hearing Impaired Children* (St. George's County Public Schools, Upper Marlboro, Md., 1977).

The general issue of early childhood education is covered very thoroughly in Ellis Evans' *Contemporary Influences in Early Childhood Education* (Holt, Rinehart & Winston, New York, 1975). For viewpoints on mainstreaming you should consult Michael Guralnick's *Early Intervention and the Integration of Handicapped and Non-Handicapped Children* (University Park Press, Baltimore, Md., 1978).

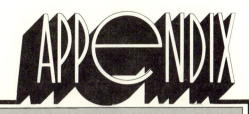

APPENDIX

○ A TEACHER'S KIT

○ B CHECK LIST FOR HEARING AIDS

○ C VIBROTACTILE AIDS

○ D SUGGESTED HANDOUTS FOR PARENTS

   1. explaining the process of hearing
   2. explaining how the cochlea works
   3. explaining conductive hearing impairment
   4. explaining sensorineural hearing impairment
   5. explaining the audiogram
   6. explaining speech in relation to the audiogram
   7. explaining degree of hearing loss
   8. explaining hearing aids
   9. explaining why hearing aids help some children more than others

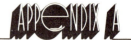

○ TEACHER'S KIT

The following items are essential for proper audiological management and should be available to the teacher at all times. (See Chapter
Seven.)

1. A listening stethoscope for listening to hearing aids.
2. A battery tester for checking batteries.
3. Pipe cleaners for cleaning earmolds.
4. An air blower for drying earmolds.
5. Spare batteries (and cords and receivers if used).
6. Scissors and double-sided adhesive tape (for example, toupé tape) for an-
   choring behind-the-ear aids.
7. A set of jewelers' screw drivers for adjusting hearing aids.
8. An otoscope to check for accumulation of wax and debris in the ear canal.

The first six items should also be included in a parent's kit.

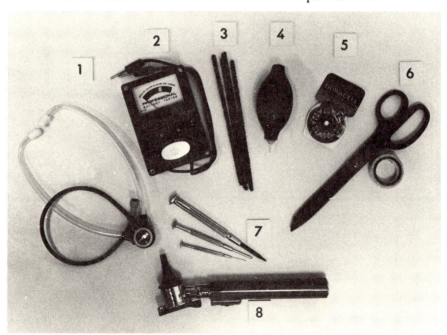

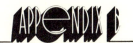

○ CHECK LIST FOR HEARING AID MONITORING

To be used by parents and teachers until routine becomes second nature. (See Chapter Seven.)

Date	Physical Condition of Aid	Physical Condition of Earmold	Listening with Stethoscope	Check for Internal Feedback	Battery Test	Comments

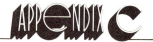

○ VIBROTACTILE AIDS

For the totally deaf child, a *vibrotactile* hearing aid can be fashioned from a higher power, body-type hearing aid and a bone conduction receiver. You should note the following, however:

1. The aid must have an excellent low frequency response.
2. The bone conductor must be matched to the hearing aid in terms of its electrical characteristics.
3. Some means must be found of keeping the vibrator in contact with the skin. I have used velcro, attached by epoxy cement, to hold the vibrator in a small hand-worn mitten.
4. This arrangement will provide very little help in most listening situations because of the interfering effects of background noise (try it yourself). In quiet rooms, however, and especially in one-to-one teaching situations, it may provide some help to the deaf child as a supplement to lipreading.
5. Deaf children cannot learn to hear with their skin.

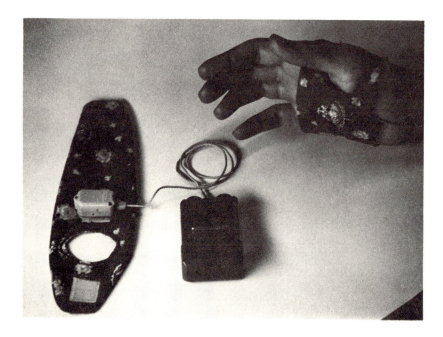

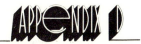
○ SOME SUGGESTED HANDOUTS FOR PARENTS

1. explaining the process of hearing

1. The *visible ear* collects sound vibrations and funnels them into the ear canal.
2. The *ear canal* passes the sound vibrations to the ear drum.
3. The *ear drum* vibrates, thus passing the sound vibrations to the middle ear.
4. The *ossicles* are three tiny bones that form a bridge to carry sound vibrations across the middle ear space.
5. The *eustachian tube* connects the middle ear space to the back of the nose. It opens periodically to let air in or out, thus preserving the correct pressure in the middle ear so that the ear drum can vibrate freely.
6. The *cochlea* is a complicated chamber filled with fluid. It receives sound vibrations from the ossicles and converts them into patterns of nerve impulses.
7. The *auditory nerve* carries the patterns of nerve impulses to the brain.
8. That part of the *brain* concerned with hearing interprets the patterns of nerve impulses and figures out what caused the original sound vibrations.

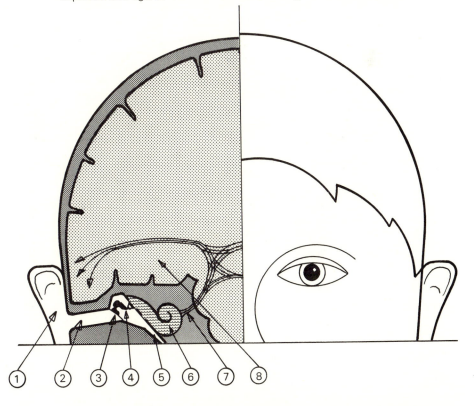

2. explaining how the cochlea works

The *cochlea* is a fluid filled tube, coiled like a snail shell and embedded in bone. It contains many membranes, nerve fibers, blood vessels and specialized cells. Sound vibrations from the ossicles pass into the cochlea and cause vibrations of the fluids and membranes.

1. The *basilar membrane* moves up and down in response to sound.
2. The *organ of corti* is attached to the basilar membrane.
3. Embedded in the organ of corti are some 16,000 *hair cells.*
4. The hairs on the hair cells are embedded in the *tectorial membrane.* Up and down movements of the basilar membrane cause the hairs to bend, thus triggering electrical impulses in the hair cells.
5. These impulses are carried to the brain along 30,000 *nerve fibers.*

This complete mechanism is about the same size as an aspirin tablet.

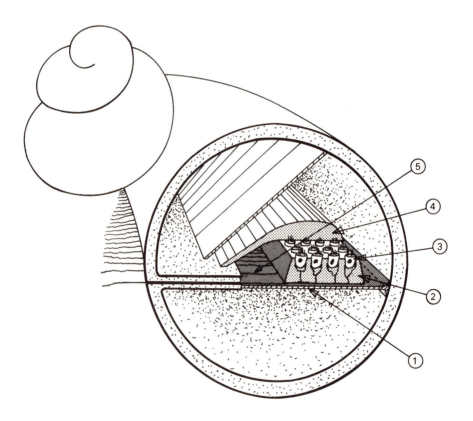

3. explaining conductive hearing impairment

Conductive hearing impairments occur when sound vibrations cannot get from the surrounding air to the fluids of the inner ear as efficiently as they should. These impairments are caused by such things as

1. Faulty development of the outer and middle ear.
2. Blockage of the ear canal (for example by wax).
3. Damage to the eardrum.
4. Damage to the ossicles.
5. Failure of the eustachian tube to let air into the middle ear cavity.
6. Collection of fluid in the middle ear cavity.
7. Infection of the middle ear cavity.
8. Growth of cysts in the middle ear cavity.
9. Growth of extra bone around the ossicles.

Conductive impairments never cause a total hearing loss, but they do cause a loss of loudness. Although many sounds may become too quiet to be heard, those that are heard sound clear and undistorted.

Most conductive impairments can be cured by medication or by surgery. Those that cannot be cured can be alleviated by hearing aids. The effect of the hearing aids is to restore the missing loudness.

Children who keep getting conductive hearing losses because of repeated ear infections may develop serious learning difficulties and perform badly in school.

4. explaining sensorineural hearing impairment

Sensorineural hearing impairments occur when the nerves of the inner ear fail to respond to sound or the hearing nerve fails to carry information to the brain. These impairments are caused by such things as

1. Faulty development of the inner ear.
2. Inherited weaknesses of the inner ear.
3. Damage to the inner ear and/or the hearing nerve from illness, drugs, or oxygen deprivation.
4. Damage to the inner ear from loud noises.

Sensorineural hearing impairments can have any degree of severity. In extreme cases the hearing loss is total. These hearing impairments cause a loss of loudness. They also cause a loss of clarity in those sounds that are loud enough to be heard.

Sensorineural hearing impairments cannot be cured by medication or surgery, but most can be alleviated, at least partially, by hearing aids. Unfortunately, however, the hearing aids only restore the missing loudness. They cannot restore the missing clarity.

Children with serious sensorineural hearing impairments have difficulty learning speech and language and, therefore, require special educational treatment.

5. explaining the audiogram

The audiogram is a chart on which we can represent sounds. Quiet sounds are represented near the top, loud sounds near the bottom. Low pitched sounds (that is deep sounds) are represented towards the left side, high pitched sounds (that is squeaky sounds) towards the right. At the very top, labelled OdB, are sounds that are only just audible to a person with normal hearing. At the very bottom are sounds that are so loud as to be painful and dangerous (even to a deaf person). Sounds at the extreme right or extreme left of the audiogram are not very informative. This leaves an area in which sounds are neither too loud, too quite, too low, or too high. This, in effect, is the area of *normal hearing*.

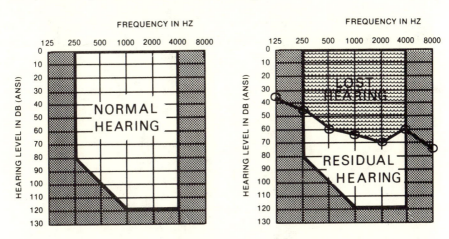

When testing someone's hearing we determine the quietest sounds he or she can hear, using tones at several pitches. The results are marked on the chart, using an O for the right ear and an X for the left, and joined by a line. This gives the individual's audiogram. The line divides the area of normal hearing into two regions. Above the line is the area of *lost hearing*. Below the line is the area of *residual hearing*.

6. explaining speech in relation to the audiogram

To developing children the most important sounds are those of conversational speech. By listening to other people's speech, they will eventually learn to understand what people say. By listening to their own speech, they will eventually learn to talk for themselves.

Speech is a complicated sound pattern that changes from moment to moment. It contains a mixture of tones—each with a different pitch. Some sounds contain mostly low pitches (for example, *m*). Some contain mostly high pitches (for example, *s*). Others contain low and high pitches in roughly equal amounts (for example, *ee*). Research has shown that the most important pitches are those whose frequencies lie between 250 Hz and 4000 Hz on the audiogram form.

The loudness of speech also changes from moment to moment. Some sounds are very quiet (for example, *f*). Other sounds are very loud (for example, *ah*). Research has shown that the tones in conversational speech fluctuate in loudness between 30dB and 60dB on the audiogram form.

With this information we can draw a *SPEECH AREA* on the audiogram form.

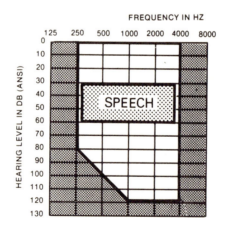

7. explaining degrees of hearing loss

The effect of a hearing loss is largely determined by the way it affects the audibility of conversational speech. For example,

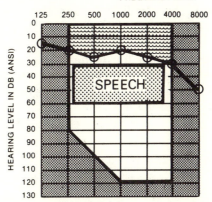

Even without hearing aids, children with *mild* hearing losses (30dB or less) have full audibility of conversational speech. Speech and language develop almost normally.

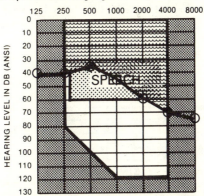

Without hearing aids, children with *moderate* hearing losses (31dB to 60dB) can hear only the louder sounds of speech. Speech and language develop spontaneously, but slowly and imperfectly.

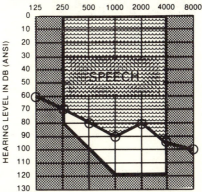

Without hearing aids, children with *severe, profound* and *total* hearing losses (greater than 60dB) do not hear normal conversational speech. Speech and language do not develop spontaneously and without proper intervention these children become functionally *deaf*.

8. explaining hearing aids

A hearing aid is like a small public address system. It picks up sound patterns with a microphone, amplifies the sound electronically, and then feeds the amplified sound into the user's ear canal. By increasing loudness, the hearing aid makes it possible for the hearing-impaired person to detect sounds that might otherwise be inaudible. Thus, the aided hearing loss is less than the unaided hearing loss. The difference between the two hearing losses is the *gain* of the hearing aid.

Several factors conspire to limit the usefulness of hearing aids:

1. The hearing aid *only* makes sound louder. If the user has a sensorineural hearing impairment, the amplified sound will lack clarity. There is nothing the hearing aid can do to restore the lost clarity.

2. The hearing aid cannot be selective. It amplifies unwanted noise just as effectively as it amplifies meaningful sounds.

3. The sounds coming out of the hearing aid may be just as loud, and therefore as uncomfortable, to a person with a sensorineural impairment, as they would be to a person with normal hearing.

4. For practical reasons we cannot provide more than about 60dB of gain.

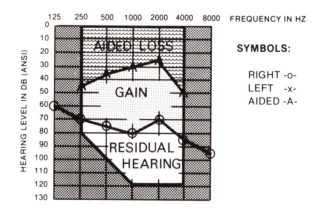

9. explaining why hearing aids help some children more than others

The usefulness of a hearing aid to a child with a sensorineural hearing impairment depends largely on the amount of residual hearing.

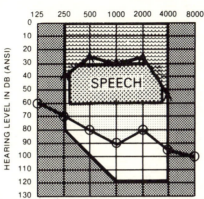

Using hearing aids, children with *severe* hearing losses (61 to 90dB) can obtain almost full audibility of conversational speech. With proper intervention such children can become functionally *hard-of hearing*.

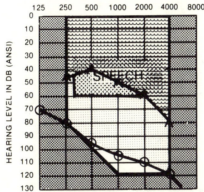

Hearing aids can provide only partial audibility of conversational speech to children with *profound* hearing losses (91 to 120dB). Nevertheless, with proper intervention, hearing can play a major role in the speech and language development of such children.

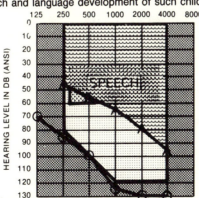

When the hearing loss is *total* (in excess of 120 dB) hearing aids obviously cannot make speech audible. The child may, however, detect speech by feeling the vibrations caused by the louder vowels.

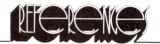

BOOTHROYD, A., "Speech Perception and Sensorineural Hearing Loss," in *Auditory Management of Hearing Impaired Children,* eds. M. Ross and T. G. Giolas. University Park Press, Baltimore, Md., 1978.

CALVERT, D. R. and S. R. SILVERMAN, *Speech and Deafness.* A. G. Bell Association for the Deaf, Washington, D.C., 1975.

COLE, P. R. and M. L. WOOD, "Differential Diagnosis," in *Pediatric Audiology,* ed. F. N. Martin. Prentice-Hall, Inc., Englewood Cliffs, N.J., 1978.

CRAIG, G. J., *Human Development.* Prentice-Hall, Inc., Englewood Cliffs, N.J., 1976.

CRITCHLEY, E., *Speech Origins and Development.* Chas. C Thomas, Springfield, Ill., 1967.

DEUTSCH, L. J. and A. M. RICHARDS, *Elementary Hearing Science.* University Park Press, Baltimore, Md., 1979.

DE VILLIERS, P. A. and J. G. DE VILLIERS, *Language Acquisition.* Harvard University Press, Cambridge, Mass., 1978.

DE VILLIERS, P. A. and J. G. DE VILLIERS, *Early Language.* Harvard University Press, Cambridge, Mass., 1979.

EISENBERG, R. B., *Auditory Competence in Early Life.* University Park Press, Baltimore, Md., 1976.

ELWOOD, P. C., W. L., JOHNSON and J. A. MANDELL, *Parent-Centered Programs for Young Hearing Impaired Children.* Prince George's County Public Schools, Upper Marlboro, Md., 1977.

ERIKSON, E. H., *Childhood and Society,* W. W. Norton & Co., Inc., New York, 1963.

EVANS, E. D., *Contemporary Influences in Early Childhood Education.* Holt, Rinehart & Winston, New York, 1975.

EWING, A. W. G. and E. C. EWING, *Teaching Deaf Children to Talk.* Manchester University Press, Manchester, U.K., 1964.

EWING, A. W. G. and E. C. EWING, *Hearing Impaired Children Under Five.* Manchester University Press, Manchester, U.K., 1971.

FRAIBERG, S. H., *The Magic Years.* Scribners, New York, 1959.

FRY, D. B., "The Role and Primacy of the Auditory Channel in Speech and Language Development," in *Auditory Management of Hearing Impaired Children,* eds. M. Ross and T. G. Giolas. University Park Press, Baltimore, Md., 1978.

GORDON, T., *Parent Effectiveness Training.* Peter H. Wyden, Inc., New York, 1970.

GREGORY, S., *The Deaf Child and His Family.* John Wiley, New York, 1976.

GRIFFITHS, C., *Conquering Childhood Deafness.* Exposition Press, New York, 1967.

GURALNICK, M. J., *Early Intervention and the Integration of Handicapped and Non-Handicapped Children.* University Park Press, Baltimore, Md., 1978.

HENEGAR, M. E. and R. O. CORNETT, *Cued Speech—Handbook for Parents.* Gallaudet College, Washington, D.C., 1971.

HORTON, K. B., "Infant Intervention and Language Learning" in *Language Perspectives,* eds. R. L. Schiefelbusch and L. L. Lloyd. University Park Press, Baltimore, Md., 1974.

HUIZING, H. C., "Auditory Training," *Acta Otolaryngologica,* Supplement 100, 1951.

JAFFE, B. F., ed., *Hearing Loss in Children.* University Park Press, Baltimore, Md., 1977.

KABAN, B., *Choosing Toys for Children.* Schocken Books, New York, 1979.

KRETSCHMER, R. R. and L. KRETSCHMER, *Language Development and Intervention with the Hearing Impaired Child.* University Park Press, Baltimore, Md., 1978.

KÜBLER-ROSS, E., *On Death and Dying.* Macmillan, New York, 1969.

LING, D., *Speech and the Hearing Impaired Child.* A. G. Bell Association for the Deaf, Washington, D.C., 1976.

LING, D., "Auditory Coding and Recoding" in *Auditory Management of Hearing Impaired Children,* eds. M. Ross and T. G. Giolas. University Park Press, Baltimore, Md., 1978.

LING, D. and M. MILNE, "The Development of Speech in Hearing-Impaired Children," in *Amplification in Education,* ed. F. H. Bess. A. G. Bell Association for the Deaf, Washington, D.C., 1981.

LUTERMAN, D., *Counselling Parents of Hearing-Impaired Children.* Little, Brown, Boston, Mass. 1979.

MACCOBY, E. E., *Social Development, Psychological Growth and the Parent-Child Relationship.* Harcourt Brace Jovanovich, Inc., New York, 1980.

MAGNER, M. E., "Techniques of Teaching" in *Speech for the Deaf Child.* ed. L. E. Connor. A. G. Bell Association for the Deaf, Washington, D.C., 1971.

MARTIN, F. N., *Introduction to Audiology,* second edition, Prentice-Hall, Inc., Englewood Cliffs, N.J., 1981.

MARTIN, F. N., ed., *Pediatric Audiology.* Prentice-Hall, Inc., Englewood Cliffs, N.J., 1978.

MENYUK, P., *Acquisition and Development of Language.* Prentice-Hall, Inc., Englewood Cliffs, N.J., 1971.

MENYUK, P., *Language and Maturation.* M.I.T. Press, Cambridge, Mass., 1977.

MERSON, R. M., B. V. FISHMAN, and S. A. FOWLER, *Central Institute Test Evaluation Booklet.* Central Institute for the Deaf, St. Louis, Mo., 1976.

MINIFIE, F. D., T. J. HIXON, and F. WILLIAMS, *Normal Aspects of Speech, Hearing and Language.* Prentice-Hall, Inc., Englewood Cliffs, N.J., 1973.

Moores, D. F., *Educating the Deaf: Psychology, Principles, and Practices.* Houghton Mifflin Co., Boston, Mass., 1978.

Murphy, A. T., ed., "The Families of Hearing Impaired Children," *Volta Review,* 81, no. 5, 1979.

Myklebust, H. R., *Your Deaf Child.* Chas. C Thomas, Springfield, Ill., 1950.

Myklebust, H. R., *Auditory Disorders in Children.* Grune & Stratton, New York, 1954.

Myklebust, H. R., *The Psychology of Deafness.* Grune & Stratton, New York, 1964.

Northcott, W. N., *Curriculum Guide: Hearing Impaired Children (0–3yrs.) and Their Parents.* A. G. Bell Association for the Deaf, Washington, D.C., 1977.

Northern, J. L. and M. Downs, *Hearing in Children* (2nd ed.). Williams & Wilkins, Baltimore, Md., 1978.

Piaget, J., and B. Inhelder, *The Psychology of the Child.* Basic Books, New York, 1969.

Pollack, D., *Educational Audiology for the Limited Hearing Infant.* Chas. C Thomas, Springfield, Ill., 1970.

Quigley, S. P., "Effects of Early Hearing Impairment on Normal Language Development" in *Pediatric Audiology,* ed. F. N. Martin. Prentice-Hall, Inc., Englewood Cliffs, N.J., 1978.

Sanders, D. A., *Aural Rehabilitation.* Prentice-Hall, Inc., Englewood Cliffs, N.J., 1971.

Sanders, D. A., *Auditory Perception of Speech.* Prentice-Hall, Inc., Englewood Cliffs, N.J., 1977.

Schlesinger, H. S. and K. P. Meadow, *Sound and Sign.* University of California Press, Berkeley, 1972.

Simmons-Martin, A., "Early Management Procedures for the Hearing Impaired Child," in *Pediatric Audiology,* ed. F. N. Martin. Prentice-Hall, Inc., Englewood Cliffs, N.J., 1978.

Simmons-Martin, A. and D. R. Calvert, eds., *Parent-Infant Intervention.* Grune & Stratton, New York, 1979.

Taylor, I. G., *Neurological Mechanisms of Speech and Hearing in Children.* Manchester University Press, Manchester, U.K., 1964.

Tiffany, W. R. and J. Carrell, *Phonetics—Theory and Application.* McGraw-Hill, New York, 1977.

Tracy Clinic, *Tracy Correspondence Course for Parents.* Tracy Clinic, Los Angeles, 1964.

Vorce, E., "Speech Curriculum," in *Speech for the Deaf Child,* ed. L. E. Connor. A. G. Bell Association for the Deaf, Washington, D.C., 1971.

Vorce, E., *Teaching Speech to Deaf Children.* A. G. Bell Association for the Deaf, Washington, D.C., 1974.

Wedenberg, E., "Auditory Training of Deaf and Hard-of-Hearing Children," *Acta Otolaryngologica,* Supplement 94, 1951.

WEDENBERG, E., "Auditory Training of Severely Hard-of-Hearing Pre-School Children," *Acta Otolaryngologica,* Supplement 110, 1954.

WHALEY, L. F., *Understanding Inherited Disorders.* C. V. Mosby, St. Louis, Mo., 1974.

WHETNALL, E. and D. B. FRY, *The Deaf Child.* Chas. C Thomas, Springfield, Ill., 1971.

WHITE, B. L. *The First Three Years.* Prentice-Hall, Inc., Englewood Cliffs, N.J., 1975.

*Page numbers in *italics* refer to tables and/or figures.